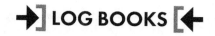 **LOG BOOKS**

THIS LOG BOOK BELONGS TO:

Name:
....

Company:
....

Establishment:
....

Address:
....

....

....

Phone:
....

Fax:
....

Email:
....

LOG BOOK START & END DATE:

Log Book Number:
....

Log Book Start Date:
....

Log Book End Date:
....

Log Book Notes:
....

....

....

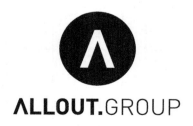

ALLOUT.GROUP

www.**ALLOUT**GROUP.co.uk

CARE HOME BEDROOM CLEANING *Checklist*

Building	Location	Room Number	Area

Start Date & Time	Finnish Date & Time	Name	Signature

	Care Home Cleaning Tasks - Bedrooms	M	T	W	T	F	S	S	Cleaned By	Checked By	Date/Time
1	Clean And Sanitize All The Desks And Tables										
2	Clean And Sanitize All The Counter Tops And Surface Areas										
3	Wipe Down The Walls Wherever There Are Spills And Splashes										
4	Disinfect Touch Points, Light Switches And Other Switches										
5	Clean And Disinfect All Doors, Handles And Doorknobs										
6	Clean And Dust Door Frames, Remember To Dust The Tops										
7	Dust Light Fixtures With A Duster Or A Microfibre Cloth										
8	Clean & Wipe Mirrors Remove Fingerprints, Smears & Dirt										
9	Clean And Dust Bedside Cabinets										
10	Clean And Sanitize Over Chair Tables										
11	Clean And Sanitize Over Bed Tables										
12	Clean And Check Bed Frames										
13	Mattresses Hoovered And Cleaned With Disinfectant										
14	Clean And Polish Bookshelves, Remember To Dust The Top										
15	Remove, Wash And Clean Any Dirty Cups Or Glasses										
16	Remove, Wash And Clean Any Dirty Plates, Bowels Or Cutlery										
17	Clean And Sanitize Any Chairs And Seats										
18	Water Jug (Washed Thoroughly Each Day & Re-Filled)										
19	Water Any Plants And Flowers										
20	Dust Plant Leafs (A Healthy Plant Needs To Be Clear Of Dust)										
21	Empty The Waste Basket And Recycling Bin										
22	Clean And Disinfectant The Waste Bin And Recycling Bin										
23	Clean And Wipe Down Windowsills										
24	Spray Air Freshener This Keeps The Room Smelling Fresh										
25	Clean And Disinfect Cabinets And Units										
26	Clean And Sanitize Desk Accessories										
27	Replace Dirty Linen And Move To Laundry Room										
28	Polish Any Wooden Furniture And Hardwood Surfaces										
29	Clean Skirting Boards/Baseboards And Corners										

Care Home Cleaning Tasks - Bedrooms Continued	M	T	W	T	F	S	S	Cleaned By	Checked By	Date/Time
Dust Television, Top Sides And Back, TV Unit And TV Stand										
Clean TV Screen With Soft Damp Cloth (Use Water/Cleaner)										
Vacuum/Hoover Between Bedroom Furniture And The Walls										
Clean And Sanitize Resident's Personal Wheelchair										
Check For Broken Wheelchairs, Frames and Wheels										
Vacuum Under Furniture, Beds, Sofas and Dressers										
Vacuum And Hoover The Carpets, Mats And Rugs										
Vacuum Furnishings, Cushions, Chairs, Sofas And Couches										
Steam Clean Carpets And Rugs										
Dust And Clean Any Picture Frames And Photo Frames										
Ledges, Flat Surfaces And The Tops Of Wardrobes Dusted										
Clean & Check Contents Of Medicine Trolleys & Cupboards										
Clean And Sanitize Mobile Phone, Phone Case And Screen										
Clean & Vacuum The Desk Chair, Legs And Chair Wheels										
Wash And Clean Air Vents										
Dust Ceiling Fan Blades With Duster Or A Microfibre Cloth										
Wash And Clean Windows (Inside And Outside)										
Dust And Clean The Walls From Top To Bottom										
Clean Blinds (Dust The Blinds With A Damp Microfibre Cloth)										
Clean Curtains (Vacuum On A Low Setting Or Wash If Possible)										
Dust And Wash Radiator Covers										
Wash And Clean Ceiling Light Covers										
Clean & Vacuum Central Heating Units (Backs Of Radiators)										
Clean And Disinfect Any Handrails										
Hand Towels Replaced With Fresh Clean Ones										
Sink Wall Mirror Cleaned With Glass Cleaner										
Sinks, Taps And Fixtures Cleaned And Disinfected										
Pour Drain Cleaner Down Sink Drains										
Check For Broken Furniture (Report/Schedule Maintenance)										
Light Bulbs Checked And None Functioning Bulbs Replaced										
Check Hardware, Door Stops And Lock Mechanisms										
Fire Exit Lights And Emergency Lights Checked & Functioning										
Test Carbon Monoxide Alarm And Replace Batteries If Required										
Test Smoke Detector Alarm And Replace Batteries If Required										
Paper Dispensers And Paper Towel Rolls Re-Stocked										
Soap Dispensers, Hand Sanitizers And Hand Gels Are Refilled										
Face Masks, Protective Gloves And Face Shields Re-Stocked										

CARE HOME COMMUNAL AREA CLEANING *Checklist*

Building	Location	Room Number	Area

Start Date & Time	Finnish Date & Time	Name	Signature

	Care Home Cleaning Tasks - Communal Area	M	T	W	T	F	S	S	Cleaned By	Checked By	Date/Time
1	Clean And Sanitize All The Desks And Tables										
2	Clean And Sanitize All The Counter Tops And Surface Areas										
3	Wipe Down The Walls Wherever There Are Spills And Splashes										
4	Disinfect Touch Points, Light Switches And Other Switches										
5	Clean And Disinfect All Doors, Handles And Doorknobs										
6	Clean And Dust Door Frames, Remember To Dust The Tops										
7	Dust Light Fixtures & Shades With A Duster Or A Microfibre Cloth										
8	Clean And Wipe Mirrors Remove Fingerprints, Smears & Dirt										
9	Clean And Sanitize Over Chair Tables										
10	Clean And Polish Bookshelves, Remember To Dust The Top										
11	Remove, Wash And Clean Any Dirty Cups Or Glasses										
12	Remove, Wash And Clean Any Dirty Plates, Bowels Or Cutlery										
13	Clean And Sanitize Any Chairs, Seats And Benches										
14	Water Jugs (Washed Thoroughly Each Day & Re-Filled)										
15	Water Any Plants And Flowers										
16	Dust Plant Leafs (A Healthy Plant Needs To Be Clear Of Dust)										
17	Empty The Waste Baskets And Recycling Bins										
18	Clean And Disinfectant The Waste Bins And Recycling Bins										
19	Clean And Wipe Down Windowsills										
20	Spray Air Freshener This Keeps The Room Smelling Fresh										
21	Clean And Disinfect Cabinets And Units										
22	Clean And Sanitize Desk Accessories										
23	Replace Dirty Table Linen And Move To Laundry Room										
24	Polish Any Wooden Furniture And Hardwood Surfaces										
25	Clean Skirting Boards/Baseboards And Corners										
26	Clean And Polish Fireplace Mantelpiece And Surrounds										
27	Wipe Down Equipment & Sanitize Tea And Coffee Making Facilities										
28	Clean And Sanitize Telephones, Cords/Leads & All Touch Points										
29	Clean And Sanitize Walking Sticks And Any Other Walking Aids										

Care Home Cleaning Tasks - Communal Area	M	T	W	T	F	S	S	Cleaned By	Checked By	Date/Time
Dust Television, Top Sides And Back, TV Unit And TV Stand										
Clean TV Screen With Soft Damp Cloth (Use Water/Cleaner)										
Vacuum/Hoover Between Furniture And The Walls										
Clean And Sanitize All Wheelchairs										
Check For Broken Wheelchairs, Frames and Wheels										
Vacuum Under Furniture, Units, Tables And Cabinets										
Vacuum And Hoover The Carpets, Mats And Rugs										
Vacuum Furnishings, Cushions, Chairs, Sofas And Couches										
Steam Clean Carpets And Rugs										
Dust And Clean Any Picture Frames And Wall Art										
Clean & Check Contents Of Medicine Trolleys & Cupboards										
Clean & Vacuum The Desk Chair, Legs And Chair Wheels										
Wash And Clean Air Vents										
Dust Ceiling Fan Blades With Duster Or A Microfibre Cloth										
Wash And Clean Windows (Inside And Outside)										
Dust And Clean The Walls From Top To Bottom										
Clean Blinds (Dust The Blinds With A Damp Microfibre Cloth)										
Clean Curtains (Vacuum On A Low Setting Or Wash If Possible)										
Dust And Wash Radiator Covers										
Wash And Clean Ceiling Light Covers										
Clean & Vacuum Central Heating Units (Backs Of Radiators)										
Clean And Disinfect Any Handrails										
Clean And Sanitize Computer, Keyboard And Computer Mice										
Clean And Sanitize iPads, Tablets, Laptops & Mobile Phones										
Floors Mopped Clean With Cleaning Or Disinfecting Solution										
The Floors Are Swept And Free From Debris And Litter										
Clean Sliding Doors and Room Partitions										
Throw Away Outdated Newspapers, Magazines, Papers										
Check For Broken Furniture (Report/Schedule Maintenance)										
Light Bulbs Checked And None Functioning Bulbs Replaced										
Check Hardware, Door Stops And Lock Mechanisms										
Fire Exit Lights And Emergency Lights Checked & Functioning										
Test Carbon Monoxide Alarm And Replace Batteries If Required										
Test Smoke Detector Alarm And Replace Batteries If Required										
Paper Dispensers And Paper Towel Rolls Re-Stocked										
Soap Dispensers, Hand Sanitizers And Hand Gels Are Refilled										
Face Masks, Protective Gloves And Face Shields Re-Stocked										

CARE HOME TOILET & RESTROOM CLEANING *Checklist*

Building	Location	Room Number	Area

Start Date & Time	Finnish Date & Time	Name	Signature

	Care Home Cleaning Tasks - Toilet & Restroom	M	T	W	T	F	S	S	Cleaned By	Checked By	Date/Time
1	Clean And Sanitize All The Counter Tops And Surface Areas										
2	Wipe Down The Walls Wherever There Are Spills And Splashes										
3	Disinfect Touch Points, Light Switches And Other Switches										
4	Clean And Disinfect All Doors, Handles And Doorknobs										
5	Clean And Dust Door Frames, Remember To Dust The Tops										
6	Dust Light Fixtures With A Duster Or A Microfibre Cloth										
7	Wall Mirrors Cleaned With Glass Cleaner										
8	Clean Any Bathroom Glasses And Cups										
9	Clean And Sanitize Any Chairs And Seats										
10	Empty The Waste Basket And Recycling Bin										
11	Clean And Disinfectant The Waste Bin And Recycling Bin										
12	Clean And Wipe Down Windowsills										
13	Spray Air Freshener This Keeps The Room Smelling Fresh										
14	Air/Odour Control Systems Are Filled And Operating Correctly										
15	Clean Skirting Boards/Baseboards And Corners										
16	Vacuum And Hoover Bath Mats, Shower Mats And Rugs										
17	Replace Bath Mats, Shower Mats And Rugs With Clean Ones										
18	Steam Clean Carpets And Rugs										
19	Hand Towels Replaced With Fresh Clean Ones										
20	Bath Towels Replaced With Fresh Clean Ones										
21	Face Towels Replaced With Fresh Clean Ones										
22	Electric Hand Dryers Cleaned, Disinfected & Operating Correctly										
23	Soap Dispensers, Sanitizers And Hand Gels Are Refilled										
24	Clean & Check Contents Of Medicine Trolleys & Cupboards										
25	Clean And Disinfect Any Handrails										
26	Sinks, Taps And Fixtures Cleaned And Disinfected										
27	Clean And Disinfect Cabinets And Units										
28	Feminine Hygiene Dispensers Re-Stocked										
29	Feminine Hygiene Bins/Containers Emptied And Cleared										

Care Home Cleaning Tasks - Toilet & Restroom	M	T	W	T	F	S	S	Cleaned By	Checked By	Date/Time
Clean & Vacuum Central Heating Units (Backs Of Radiators)										
Wash And Clean Ceiling Light Covers										
Toilet Roll Holders And Toilet Rolls Re-Stocked										
Toilet Roll Holders Cleaned And Disinfected										
Clean Inside The Toilets And Urinals With Disinfectant										
Toilet Seats Cleaned And Disinfected										
Clean Top Of Toilets Tanks, The Bases And Behind Toilets										
Urinal Handles Cleaned And Disinfected										
Urinal Screens Cleaned, Disinfected And Blocks Replaced										
Paper Dispensers And Paper Towel Rolls Re-Stocked										
Paper Dispensers And Paper Towel Roll Cleaned & Disinfected										
The Floors Are Swept And Free From Debris And Litter										
Floors Mopped Clean With Cleaning Or Disinfecting Solution										
Put Up Or Place Wet Floor Signs After Mopping Floors										
Showers And Shower Heads, Cleaned And Disinfected										
Soak Shower Heads										
Clean And Disinfect Glass Shower Doors/Outer Doors										
Clean Soap Scum From Shower Walls										
Clean Blinds (Dust The Blinds With A Damp Microfibre Cloth)										
Clean Curtains (Vacuum On A Low Setting Or Wash If Possible)										
Dust And Wash Radiator Covers										
Clean And Disinfect Commodes Between Each Use										
Clean And Disinfect Shower Chairs Between Each Use										
Bath Hoists Cleaned And Disinfected Between Each Use										
Scrub Tub/Bath, Polish Facets And Taps, Clean & Disinfected										
Toothbrush Holders And Soap Holders Cleaned										
Re-Place Shower Curtains With Clean Fresh Ones										
Wash And Clean Air Vents										
Thoroughly Clean Grout And Tiles										
Disinfect And Clean All The Walls From Top To Bottom										
Wash And Clean Windows (Inside And Outside)										
Unclog The Drains (Sink, Bath And Shower)										
Pour Drain Cleaner Down Sink, Shower & Bath Drains										
Floor Drains And Drain Covers Are Open And Free Of Debris										
Hair Dryers Cleaned And Disinfected And Operating Correctly										
Light Bulbs Checked And None Functioning Bulbs Replaced										
Check Hardware, Door Stops And Lock Mechanisms										

CARE HOME BEDROOM CLEANING *Checklist*

Building	Location	Room Number	Area

Start Date & Time	Finnish Date & Time	Name	Signature

	Care Home Cleaning Tasks - Bedrooms	M	T	W	T	F	S	S	Cleaned By	Checked By	Date/Time
1	Clean And Sanitize All The Desks And Tables										
2	Clean And Sanitize All The Counter Tops And Surface Areas										
3	Wipe Down The Walls Wherever There Are Spills And Splashes										
4	Disinfect Touch Points, Light Switches And Other Switches										
5	Clean And Disinfect All Doors, Handles And Doorknobs										
6	Clean And Dust Door Frames, Remember To Dust The Tops										
7	Dust Light Fixtures With A Duster Or A Microfibre Cloth										
8	Clean & Wipe Mirrors Remove Fingerprints, Smears & Dirt										
9	Clean And Dust Bedside Cabinets										
10	Clean And Sanitize Over Chair Tables										
11	Clean And Sanitize Over Bed Tables										
12	Clean And Check Bed Frames										
13	Mattresses Hoovered And Cleaned With Disinfectant										
14	Clean And Polish Bookshelves, Remember To Dust The Top										
15	Remove, Wash And Clean Any Dirty Cups Or Glasses										
16	Remove, Wash And Clean Any Dirty Plates, Bowels Or Cutlery										
17	Clean And Sanitize Any Chairs And Seats										
18	Water Jug (Washed Thoroughly Each Day & Re-Filled)										
19	Water Any Plants And Flowers										
20	Dust Plant Leafs (A Healthy Plant Needs To Be Clear Of Dust)										
21	Empty The Waste Basket And Recycling Bin										
22	Clean And Disinfectant The Waste Bin And Recycling Bin										
23	Clean And Wipe Down Windowsills										
24	Spray Air Freshener This Keeps The Room Smelling Fresh										
25	Clean And Disinfect Cabinets And Units										
26	Clean And Sanitize Desk Accessories										
27	Replace Dirty Linen And Move To Laundry Room										
28	Polish Any Wooden Furniture And Hardwood Surfaces										
29	Clean Skirting Boards/Baseboards And Corners										

Care Home Cleaning Tasks - Bedrooms Continued	M	T	W	T	F	S	S	Cleaned By	Checked By	Date/Time
Dust Television, Top Sides And Back, TV Unit And TV Stand										
Clean TV Screen With Soft Damp Cloth (Use Water/Cleaner)										
Vacuum/Hoover Between Bedroom Furniture And The Walls										
Clean And Sanitize Resident's Personal Wheelchair										
Check For Broken Wheelchairs, Frames and Wheels										
Vacuum Under Furniture, Beds, Sofas and Dressers										
Vacuum And Hoover The Carpets, Mats And Rugs										
Vacuum Furnishings, Cushions, Chairs, Sofas And Couches										
Steam Clean Carpets And Rugs										
Dust And Clean Any Picture Frames And Photo Frames										
Ledges, Flat Surfaces And The Tops Of Wardrobes Dusted										
Clean & Check Contents Of Medicine Trolleys & Cupboards										
Clean And Sanitize Mobile Phone, Phone Case And Screen										
Clean & Vacuum The Desk Chair, Legs And Chair Wheels										
Wash And Clean Air Vents										
Dust Ceiling Fan Blades With Duster Or A Microfibre Cloth										
Wash And Clean Windows (Inside And Outside)										
Dust And Clean The Walls From Top To Bottom										
Clean Blinds (Dust The Blinds With A Damp Microfibre Cloth)										
Clean Curtains (Vacuum On A Low Setting Or Wash If Possible)										
Dust And Wash Radiator Covers										
Wash And Clean Ceiling Light Covers										
Clean & Vacuum Central Heating Units (Backs Of Radiators)										
Clean And Disinfect Any Handrails										
Hand Towels Replaced With Fresh Clean Ones										
Sink Wall Mirror Cleaned With Glass Cleaner										
Sinks, Taps And Fixtures Cleaned And Disinfected										
Pour Drain Cleaner Down Sink Drains										
Check For Broken Furniture (Report/Schedule Maintenance)										
Light Bulbs Checked And None Functioning Bulbs Replaced										
Check Hardware, Door Stops And Lock Mechanisms										
Fire Exit Lights And Emergency Lights Checked & Functioning										
Test Carbon Monoxide Alarm And Replace Batteries If Required										
Test Smoke Detector Alarm And Replace Batteries If Required										
Paper Dispensers And Paper Towel Rolls Re-Stocked										
Soap Dispensers, Hand Sanitizers And Hand Gels Are Refilled										
Face Masks, Protective Gloves And Face Shields Re-Stocked										

CARE HOME COMMUNAL AREA CLEANING *Checklist*

Building	Location	Room Number	Area

Start Date & Time	Finnish Date & Time	Name	Signature

	Care Home Cleaning Tasks - Communal Area	M	T	W	T	F	S	S	Cleaned By	Checked By	Date/Time
1	Clean And Sanitize All The Desks And Tables										
2	Clean And Sanitize All The Counter Tops And Surface Areas										
3	Wipe Down The Walls Wherever There Are Spills And Splashes										
4	Disinfect Touch Points, Light Switches And Other Switches										
5	Clean And Disinfect All Doors, Handles And Doorknobs										
6	Clean And Dust Door Frames, Remember To Dust The Tops										
7	Dust Light Fixtures & Shades With A Duster Or A Microfibre Cloth										
8	Clean And Wipe Mirrors Remove Fingerprints, Smears & Dirt										
9	Clean And Sanitize Over Chair Tables										
10	Clean And Polish Bookshelves, Remember To Dust The Top										
11	Remove, Wash And Clean Any Dirty Cups Or Glasses										
12	Remove, Wash And Clean Any Dirty Plates, Bowels Or Cutlery										
13	Clean And Sanitize Any Chairs, Seats And Benches										
14	Water Jugs (Washed Thoroughly Each Day & Re-Filled)										
15	Water Any Plants And Flowers										
16	Dust Plant Leafs (A Healthy Plant Needs To Be Clear Of Dust)										
17	Empty The Waste Baskets And Recycling Bins										
18	Clean And Disinfectant The Waste Bins And Recycling Bins										
19	Clean And Wipe Down Windowsills										
20	Spray Air Freshener This Keeps The Room Smelling Fresh										
21	Clean And Disinfect Cabinets And Units										
22	Clean And Sanitize Desk Accessories										
23	Replace Dirty Table Linen And Move To Laundry Room										
24	Polish Any Wooden Furniture And Hardwood Surfaces										
25	Clean Skirting Boards/Baseboards And Corners										
26	Clean And Polish Fireplace Mantelpiece And Surrounds										
27	Wipe Down Equipment & Sanitize Tea And Coffee Making Facilities										
28	Clean And Sanitize Telephones, Cords/Leads & All Touch Points										
29	Clean And Sanitize Walking Sticks And Any Other Walking Aids										

Care Home Cleaning Tasks - Communal Area	M	T	W	T	F	S	S	Cleaned By	Checked By	Date/Time
Dust Television, Top Sides And Back, TV Unit And TV Stand										
Clean TV Screen With Soft Damp Cloth (Use Water/Cleaner)										
Vacuum/Hoover Between Furniture And The Walls										
Clean And Sanitize All Wheelchairs										
Check For Broken Wheelchairs, Frames and Wheels										
Vacuum Under Furniture, Units, Tables And Cabinets										
Vacuum And Hoover The Carpets, Mats And Rugs										
Vacuum Furnishings, Cushions, Chairs, Sofas And Couches										
Steam Clean Carpets And Rugs										
Dust And Clean Any Picture Frames And Wall Art										
Clean & Check Contents Of Medicine Trolleys & Cupboards										
Clean & Vacuum The Desk Chair, Legs And Chair Wheels										
Wash And Clean Air Vents										
Dust Ceiling Fan Blades With Duster Or A Microfibre Cloth										
Wash And Clean Windows (Inside And Outside)										
Dust And Clean The Walls From Top To Bottom										
Clean Blinds (Dust The Blinds With A Damp Microfibre Cloth)										
Clean Curtains (Vacuum On A Low Setting Or Wash If Possible)										
Dust And Wash Radiator Covers										
Wash And Clean Ceiling Light Covers										
Clean & Vacuum Central Heating Units (Backs Of Radiators)										
Clean And Disinfect Any Handrails										
Clean And Sanitize Computer, Keyboard And Computer Mice										
Clean And Sanitize iPads, Tablets, Laptops & Mobile Phones										
Floors Mopped Clean With Cleaning Or Disinfecting Solution										
The Floors Are Swept And Free From Debris And Litter										
Clean Sliding Doors and Room Partitions										
Throw Away Outdated Newspapers, Magazines, Papers										
Check For Broken Furniture (Report/Schedule Maintenance)										
Light Bulbs Checked And None Functioning Bulbs Replaced										
Check Hardware, Door Stops And Lock Mechanisms										
Fire Exit Lights And Emergency Lights Checked & Functioning										
Test Carbon Monoxide Alarm And Replace Batteries If Required										
Test Smoke Detector Alarm And Replace Batteries If Required										
Paper Dispensers And Paper Towel Rolls Re-Stocked										
Soap Dispensers, Hand Sanitizers And Hand Gels Are Refilled										
Face Masks, Protective Gloves And Face Shields Re-Stocked										

CARE HOME TOILET & RESTROOM CLEANING *Checklist*

Building	Location	Room Number	Area

Start Date & Time	Finnish Date & Time	Name	Signature

	Care Home Cleaning Tasks - Toilet & Restroom	M	T	W	T	F	S	S	Cleaned By	Checked By	Date/Time
1	Clean And Sanitize All The Counter Tops And Surface Areas										
2	Wipe Down The Walls Wherever There Are Spills And Splashes										
3	Disinfect Touch Points, Light Switches And Other Switches										
4	Clean And Disinfect All Doors, Handles And Doorknobs										
5	Clean And Dust Door Frames, Remember To Dust The Tops										
6	Dust Light Fixtures With A Duster Or A Microfibre Cloth										
7	Wall Mirrors Cleaned With Glass Cleaner										
8	Clean Any Bathroom Glasses And Cups										
9	Clean And Sanitize Any Chairs And Seats										
10	Empty The Waste Basket And Recycling Bin										
11	Clean And Disinfectant The Waste Bin And Recycling Bin										
12	Clean And Wipe Down Windowsills										
13	Spray Air Freshener This Keeps The Room Smelling Fresh										
14	Air/Odour Control Systems Are Filled And Operating Correctly										
15	Clean Skirting Boards/Baseboards And Corners										
16	Vacuum And Hoover Bath Mats, Shower Mats And Rugs										
17	Replace Bath Mats, Shower Mats And Rugs With Clean Ones										
18	Steam Clean Carpets And Rugs										
19	Hand Towels Replaced With Fresh Clean Ones										
20	Bath Towels Replaced With Fresh Clean Ones										
21	Face Towels Replaced With Fresh Clean Ones										
22	Electric Hand Dryers Cleaned, Disinfected & Operating Correctly										
23	Soap Dispensers, Sanitizers And Hand Gels Are Refilled										
24	Clean & Check Contents Of Medicine Trolleys & Cupboards										
25	Clean And Disinfect Any Handrails										
26	Sinks, Taps And Fixtures Cleaned And Disinfected										
27	Clean And Disinfect Cabinets And Units										
28	Feminine Hygiene Dispensers Re-Stocked										
29	Feminine Hygiene Bins/Containers Emptied And Cleared										

Care Home Cleaning Tasks - Toilet & Restroom	M	T	W	T	F	S	S	Cleaned By	Checked By	Date/Time
Clean & Vacuum Central Heating Units (Backs Of Radiators)										
Wash And Clean Ceiling Light Covers										
Toilet Roll Holders And Toilet Rolls Re-Stocked										
Toilet Roll Holders Cleaned And Disinfected										
Clean Inside The Toilets And Urinals With Disinfectant										
Toilet Seats Cleaned And Disinfected										
Clean Top Of Toilets Tanks, The Bases And Behind Toilets										
Urinal Handles Cleaned And Disinfected										
Urinal Screens Cleaned, Disinfected And Blocks Replaced										
Paper Dispensers And Paper Towel Rolls Re-Stocked										
Paper Dispensers And Paper Towel Roll Cleaned & Disinfected										
The Floors Are Swept And Free From Debris And Litter										
Floors Mopped Clean With Cleaning Or Disinfecting Solution										
Put Up Or Place Wet Floor Signs After Mopping Floors										
Showers And Shower Heads, Cleaned And Disinfected										
Soak Shower Heads										
Clean And Disinfect Glass Shower Doors/Outer Doors										
Clean Soap Scum From Shower Walls										
Clean Blinds (Dust The Blinds With A Damp Microfibre Cloth)										
Clean Curtains (Vacuum On A Low Setting Or Wash If Possible)										
Dust And Wash Radiator Covers										
Clean And Disinfect Commodes Between Each Use										
Clean And Disinfect Shower Chairs Between Each Use										
Bath Hoists Cleaned And Disinfected Between Each Use										
Scrub Tub/Bath, Polish Facets And Taps, Clean & Disinfected										
Toothbrush Holders And Soap Holders Cleaned										
Re-Place Shower Curtains With Clean Fresh Ones										
Wash And Clean Air Vents										
Thoroughly Clean Grout And Tiles										
Disinfect And Clean All The Walls From Top To Bottom										
Wash And Clean Windows (Inside And Outside)										
Unclog The Drains (Sink, Bath And Shower)										
Pour Drain Cleaner Down Sink, Shower & Bath Drains										
Floor Drains And Drain Covers Are Open And Free Of Debris										
Hair Dryers Cleaned And Disinfected And Operating Correctly										
Light Bulbs Checked And None Functioning Bulbs Replaced										
Check Hardware, Door Stops And Lock Mechanisms										

CARE HOME BEDROOM CLEANING *Checklist*

Building	Location	Room Number	Area

Start Date & Time	Finnish Date & Time	Name	Signature

	Care Home Cleaning Tasks - Bedrooms	M	T	W	T	F	S	S	Cleaned By	Checked By	Date/Time
1	Clean And Sanitize All The Desks And Tables										
2	Clean And Sanitize All The Counter Tops And Surface Areas										
3	Wipe Down The Walls Wherever There Are Spills And Splashes										
4	Disinfect Touch Points, Light Switches And Other Switches										
5	Clean And Disinfect All Doors, Handles And Doorknobs										
6	Clean And Dust Door Frames, Remember To Dust The Tops										
7	Dust Light Fixtures With A Duster Or A Microfibre Cloth										
8	Clean & Wipe Mirrors Remove Fingerprints, Smears & Dirt										
9	Clean And Dust Bedside Cabinets										
10	Clean And Sanitize Over Chair Tables										
11	Clean And Sanitize Over Bed Tables										
12	Clean And Check Bed Frames										
13	Mattresses Hoovered And Cleaned With Disinfectant										
14	Clean And Polish Bookshelves, Remember To Dust The Top										
15	Remove, Wash And Clean Any Dirty Cups Or Glasses										
16	Remove, Wash And Clean Any Dirty Plates, Bowels Or Cutlery										
17	Clean And Sanitize Any Chairs And Seats										
18	Water Jug (Washed Thoroughly Each Day & Re-Filled)										
19	Water Any Plants And Flowers										
20	Dust Plant Leafs (A Healthy Plant Needs To Be Clear Of Dust)										
21	Empty The Waste Basket And Recycling Bin										
22	Clean And Disinfectant The Waste Bin And Recycling Bin										
23	Clean And Wipe Down Windowsills										
24	Spray Air Freshener This Keeps The Room Smelling Fresh										
25	Clean And Disinfect Cabinets And Units										
26	Clean And Sanitize Desk Accessories										
27	Replace Dirty Linen And Move To Laundry Room										
28	Polish Any Wooden Furniture And Hardwood Surfaces										
29	Clean Skirting Boards/Baseboards And Corners										

Care Home Cleaning Tasks - Bedrooms Continued	M	T	W	T	F	S	S	Cleaned By	Checked By	Date/Time
Dust Television, Top Sides And Back, TV Unit And TV Stand										
Clean TV Screen With Soft Damp Cloth (Use Water/Cleaner)										
Vacuum/Hoover Between Bedroom Furniture And The Walls										
Clean And Sanitize Resident's Personal Wheelchair										
Check For Broken Wheelchairs, Frames and Wheels										
Vacuum Under Furniture, Beds, Sofas and Dressers										
Vacuum And Hoover The Carpets, Mats And Rugs										
Vacuum Furnishings, Cushions, Chairs, Sofas And Couches										
Steam Clean Carpets And Rugs										
Dust And Clean Any Picture Frames And Photo Frames										
Ledges, Flat Surfaces And The Tops Of Wardrobes Dusted										
Clean & Check Contents Of Medicine Trolleys & Cupboards										
Clean And Sanitize Mobile Phone, Phone Case And Screen										
Clean & Vacuum The Desk Chair, Legs And Chair Wheels										
Wash And Clean Air Vents										
Dust Ceiling Fan Blades With Duster Or A Microfibre Cloth										
Wash And Clean Windows (Inside And Outside)										
Dust And Clean The Walls From Top To Bottom										
Clean Blinds (Dust The Blinds With A Damp Microfibre Cloth)										
Clean Curtains (Vacuum On A Low Setting Or Wash If Possible)										
Dust And Wash Radiator Covers										
Wash And Clean Ceiling Light Covers										
Clean & Vacuum Central Heating Units (Backs Of Radiators)										
Clean And Disinfect Any Handrails										
Hand Towels Replaced With Fresh Clean Ones										
Sink Wall Mirror Cleaned With Glass Cleaner										
Sinks, Taps And Fixtures Cleaned And Disinfected										
Pour Drain Cleaner Down Sink Drains										
Check For Broken Furniture (Report/Schedule Maintenance)										
Light Bulbs Checked And None Functioning Bulbs Replaced										
Check Hardware, Door Stops And Lock Mechanisms										
Fire Exit Lights And Emergency Lights Checked & Functioning										
Test Carbon Monoxide Alarm And Replace Batteries If Required										
Test Smoke Detector Alarm And Replace Batteries If Required										
Paper Dispensers And Paper Towel Rolls Re-Stocked										
Soap Dispensers, Hand Sanitizers And Hand Gels Are Refilled										
Face Masks, Protective Gloves And Face Shields Re-Stocked										

CARE HOME COMMUNAL AREA CLEANING *Checklist*

Building	Location	Room Number	Area

Start Date & Time	Finnish Date & Time	Name	Signature

	Care Home Cleaning Tasks - Communal Area	M	T	W	T	F	S	S	Cleaned By	Checked By	Date/Time
1	Clean And Sanitize All The Desks And Tables										
2	Clean And Sanitize All The Counter Tops And Surface Areas										
3	Wipe Down The Walls Wherever There Are Spills And Splashes										
4	Disinfect Touch Points, Light Switches And Other Switches										
5	Clean And Disinfect All Doors, Handles And Doorknobs										
6	Clean And Dust Door Frames, Remember To Dust The Tops										
7	Dust Light Fixtures & Shades With A Duster Or A Microfibre Cloth										
8	Clean And Wipe Mirrors Remove Fingerprints, Smears & Dirt										
9	Clean And Sanitize Over Chair Tables										
10	Clean And Polish Bookshelves, Remember To Dust The Top										
11	Remove, Wash And Clean Any Dirty Cups Or Glasses										
12	Remove, Wash And Clean Any Dirty Plates, Bowels Or Cutlery										
13	Clean And Sanitize Any Chairs, Seats And Benches										
14	Water Jugs (Washed Thoroughly Each Day & Re-Filled)										
15	Water Any Plants And Flowers										
16	Dust Plant Leafs (A Healthy Plant Needs To Be Clear Of Dust)										
17	Empty The Waste Baskets And Recycling Bins										
18	Clean And Disinfectant The Waste Bins And Recycling Bins										
19	Clean And Wipe Down Windowsills										
20	Spray Air Freshener This Keeps The Room Smelling Fresh										
21	Clean And Disinfect Cabinets And Units										
22	Clean And Sanitize Desk Accessories										
23	Replace Dirty Table Linen And Move To Laundry Room										
24	Polish Any Wooden Furniture And Hardwood Surfaces										
25	Clean Skirting Boards/Baseboards And Corners										
26	Clean And Polish Fireplace Mantelpiece And Surrounds										
27	Wipe Down Equipment & Sanitize Tea And Coffee Making Facilities										
28	Clean And Sanitize Telephones, Cords/Leads & All Touch Points										
29	Clean And Sanitize Walking Sticks And Any Other Walking Aids										

Care Home Cleaning Tasks - Communal Area	M	T	W	T	F	S	S	Cleaned By	Checked By	Date/Time
Dust Television, Top Sides And Back, TV Unit And TV Stand										
Clean TV Screen With Soft Damp Cloth (Use Water/Cleaner)										
Vacuum/Hoover Between Furniture And The Walls										
Clean And Sanitize All Wheelchairs										
Check For Broken Wheelchairs, Frames and Wheels										
Vacuum Under Furniture, Units, Tables And Cabinets										
Vacuum And Hoover The Carpets, Mats And Rugs										
Vacuum Furnishings, Cushions, Chairs, Sofas And Couches										
Steam Clean Carpets And Rugs										
Dust And Clean Any Picture Frames And Wall Art										
Clean & Check Contents Of Medicine Trolleys & Cupboards										
Clean & Vacuum The Desk Chair, Legs And Chair Wheels										
Wash And Clean Air Vents										
Dust Ceiling Fan Blades With Duster Or A Microfibre Cloth										
Wash And Clean Windows (Inside And Outside)										
Dust And Clean The Walls From Top To Bottom										
Clean Blinds (Dust The Blinds With A Damp Microfibre Cloth)										
Clean Curtains (Vacuum On A Low Setting Or Wash If Possible)										
Dust And Wash Radiator Covers										
Wash And Clean Ceiling Light Covers										
Clean & Vacuum Central Heating Units (Backs Of Radiators)										
Clean And Disinfect Any Handrails										
Clean And Sanitize Computer, Keyboard And Computer Mice										
Clean And Sanitize iPads, Tablets, Laptops & Mobile Phones										
Floors Mopped Clean With Cleaning Or Disinfecting Solution										
The Floors Are Swept And Free From Debris And Litter										
Clean Sliding Doors and Room Partitions										
Throw Away Outdated Newspapers, Magazines, Papers										
Check For Broken Furniture (Report/Schedule Maintenance)										
Light Bulbs Checked And None Functioning Bulbs Replaced										
Check Hardware, Door Stops And Lock Mechanisms										
Fire Exit Lights And Emergency Lights Checked & Functioning										
Test Carbon Monoxide Alarm And Replace Batteries If Required										
Test Smoke Detector Alarm And Replace Batteries If Required										
Paper Dispensers And Paper Towel Rolls Re-Stocked										
Soap Dispensers, Hand Sanitizers And Hand Gels Are Refilled										
Face Masks, Protective Gloves And Face Shields Re-Stocked										

CARE HOME TOILET & RESTROOM CLEANING *Checklist*

Building	Location	Room Number	Area

Start Date & Time	Finnish Date & Time	Name	Signature

	Care Home Cleaning Tasks - Toilet & Restroom	M	T	W	T	F	S	S	Cleaned By	Checked By	Date/Time
1	Clean And Sanitize All The Counter Tops And Surface Areas										
2	Wipe Down The Walls Wherever There Are Spills And Splashes										
3	Disinfect Touch Points, Light Switches And Other Switches										
4	Clean And Disinfect All Doors, Handles And Doorknobs										
5	Clean And Dust Door Frames, Remember To Dust The Tops										
6	Dust Light Fixtures With A Duster Or A Microfibre Cloth										
7	Wall Mirrors Cleaned With Glass Cleaner										
8	Clean Any Bathroom Glasses And Cups										
9	Clean And Sanitize Any Chairs And Seats										
10	Empty The Waste Basket And Recycling Bin										
11	Clean And Disinfectant The Waste Bin And Recycling Bin										
12	Clean And Wipe Down Windowsills										
13	Spray Air Freshener This Keeps The Room Smelling Fresh										
14	Air/Odour Control Systems Are Filled And Operating Correctly										
15	Clean Skirting Boards/Baseboards And Corners										
16	Vacuum And Hoover Bath Mats, Shower Mats And Rugs										
17	Replace Bath Mats, Shower Mats And Rugs With Clean Ones										
18	Steam Clean Carpets And Rugs										
19	Hand Towels Replaced With Fresh Clean Ones										
20	Bath Towels Replaced With Fresh Clean Ones										
21	Face Towels Replaced With Fresh Clean Ones										
22	Electric Hand Dryers Cleaned, Disinfected & Operating Correctly										
23	Soap Dispensers, Sanitizers And Hand Gels Are Refilled										
24	Clean & Check Contents Of Medicine Trolleys & Cupboards										
25	Clean And Disinfect Any Handrails										
26	Sinks, Taps And Fixtures Cleaned And Disinfected										
27	Clean And Disinfect Cabinets And Units										
28	Feminine Hygiene Dispensers Re-Stocked										
29	Feminine Hygiene Bins/Containers Emptied And Cleared										

Care Home Cleaning Tasks - Toilet & Restroom	M	T	W	T	F	S	S	Cleaned By	Checked By	Date/Time
Clean & Vacuum Central Heating Units (Backs Of Radiators)										
Wash And Clean Ceiling Light Covers										
Toilet Roll Holders And Toilet Rolls Re-Stocked										
Toilet Roll Holders Cleaned And Disinfected										
Clean Inside The Toilets And Urinals With Disinfectant										
Toilet Seats Cleaned And Disinfected										
Clean Top Of Toilets Tanks, The Bases And Behind Toilets										
Urinal Handles Cleaned And Disinfected										
Urinal Screens Cleaned, Disinfected And Blocks Replaced										
Paper Dispensers And Paper Towel Rolls Re-Stocked										
Paper Dispensers And Paper Towel Roll Cleaned & Disinfected										
The Floors Are Swept And Free From Debris And Litter										
Floors Mopped Clean With Cleaning Or Disinfecting Solution										
Put Up Or Place Wet Floor Signs After Mopping Floors										
Showers And Shower Heads, Cleaned And Disinfected										
Soak Shower Heads										
Clean And Disinfect Glass Shower Doors/Outer Doors										
Clean Soap Scum From Shower Walls										
Clean Blinds (Dust The Blinds With A Damp Microfibre Cloth)										
Clean Curtains (Vacuum On A Low Setting Or Wash If Possible)										
Dust And Wash Radiator Covers										
Clean And Disinfect Commodes Between Each Use										
Clean And Disinfect Shower Chairs Between Each Use										
Bath Hoists Cleaned And Disinfected Between Each Use										
Scrub Tub/Bath, Polish Facets And Taps, Clean & Disinfected										
Toothbrush Holders And Soap Holders Cleaned										
Re-Place Shower Curtains With Clean Fresh Ones										
Wash And Clean Air Vents										
Thoroughly Clean Grout And Tiles										
Disinfect And Clean All The Walls From Top To Bottom										
Wash And Clean Windows (Inside And Outside)										
Unclog The Drains (Sink, Bath And Shower)										
Pour Drain Cleaner Down Sink, Shower & Bath Drains										
Floor Drains And Drain Covers Are Open And Free Of Debris										
Hair Dryers Cleaned And Disinfected And Operating Correctly										
Light Bulbs Checked And None Functioning Bulbs Replaced										
Check Hardware, Door Stops And Lock Mechanisms										

CARE HOME BEDROOM CLEANING *Checklist*

Building	Location	Room Number	Area

Start Date & Time	Finnish Date & Time	Name	Signature

	Care Home Cleaning Tasks - Bedrooms	M	T	W	T	F	S	S	Cleaned By	Checked By	Date/Time
1	Clean And Sanitize All The Desks And Tables										
2	Clean And Sanitize All The Counter Tops And Surface Areas										
3	Wipe Down The Walls Wherever There Are Spills And Splashes										
4	Disinfect Touch Points, Light Switches And Other Switches										
5	Clean And Disinfect All Doors, Handles And Doorknobs										
6	Clean And Dust Door Frames, Remember To Dust The Tops										
7	Dust Light Fixtures With A Duster Or A Microfibre Cloth										
8	Clean & Wipe Mirrors Remove Fingerprints, Smears & Dirt										
9	Clean And Dust Bedside Cabinets										
10	Clean And Sanitize Over Chair Tables										
11	Clean And Sanitize Over Bed Tables										
12	Clean And Check Bed Frames										
13	Mattresses Hoovered And Cleaned With Disinfectant										
14	Clean And Polish Bookshelves, Remember To Dust The Top										
15	Remove, Wash And Clean Any Dirty Cups Or Glasses										
16	Remove, Wash And Clean Any Dirty Plates, Bowels Or Cutlery										
17	Clean And Sanitize Any Chairs And Seats										
18	Water Jug (Washed Thoroughly Each Day & Re-Filled)										
19	Water Any Plants And Flowers										
20	Dust Plant Leafs (A Healthy Plant Needs To Be Clear Of Dust)										
21	Empty The Waste Basket And Recycling Bin										
22	Clean And Disinfectant The Waste Bin And Recycling Bin										
23	Clean And Wipe Down Windowsills										
24	Spray Air Freshener This Keeps The Room Smelling Fresh										
25	Clean And Disinfect Cabinets And Units										
26	Clean And Sanitize Desk Accessories										
27	Replace Dirty Linen And Move To Laundry Room										
28	Polish Any Wooden Furniture And Hardwood Surfaces										
29	Clean Skirting Boards/Baseboards And Corners										

Care Home Cleaning Tasks - Bedrooms Continued	M	T	W	T	F	S	S	Cleaned By	Checked By	Date/Time
Dust Television, Top Sides And Back, TV Unit And TV Stand										
Clean TV Screen With Soft Damp Cloth (Use Water/Cleaner)										
Vacuum/Hoover Between Bedroom Furniture And The Walls										
Clean And Sanitize Resident's Personal Wheelchair										
Check For Broken Wheelchairs, Frames and Wheels										
Vacuum Under Furniture, Beds, Sofas and Dressers										
Vacuum And Hoover The Carpets, Mats And Rugs										
Vacuum Furnishings, Cushions, Chairs, Sofas And Couches										
Steam Clean Carpets And Rugs										
Dust And Clean Any Picture Frames And Photo Frames										
Ledges, Flat Surfaces And The Tops Of Wardrobes Dusted										
Clean & Check Contents Of Medicine Trolleys & Cupboards										
Clean And Sanitize Mobile Phone, Phone Case And Screen										
Clean & Vacuum The Desk Chair, Legs And Chair Wheels										
Wash And Clean Air Vents										
Dust Ceiling Fan Blades With Duster Or A Microfibre Cloth										
Wash And Clean Windows (Inside And Outside)										
Dust And Clean The Walls From Top To Bottom										
Clean Blinds (Dust The Blinds With A Damp Microfibre Cloth)										
Clean Curtains (Vacuum On A Low Setting Or Wash If Possible)										
Dust And Wash Radiator Covers										
Wash And Clean Ceiling Light Covers										
Clean & Vacuum Central Heating Units (Backs Of Radiators)										
Clean And Disinfect Any Handrails										
Hand Towels Replaced With Fresh Clean Ones										
Sink Wall Mirror Cleaned With Glass Cleaner										
Sinks, Taps And Fixtures Cleaned And Disinfected										
Pour Drain Cleaner Down Sink Drains										
Check For Broken Furniture (Report/Schedule Maintenance)										
Light Bulbs Checked And None Functioning Bulbs Replaced										
Check Hardware, Door Stops And Lock Mechanisms										
Fire Exit Lights And Emergency Lights Checked & Functioning										
Test Carbon Monoxide Alarm And Replace Batteries If Required										
Test Smoke Detector Alarm And Replace Batteries If Required										
Paper Dispensers And Paper Towel Rolls Re-Stocked										
Soap Dispensers, Hand Sanitizers And Hand Gels Are Refilled										
Face Masks, Protective Gloves And Face Shields Re-Stocked										

CARE HOME COMMUNAL AREA CLEANING *Checklist*

Building	Location	Room Number	Area

Start Date & Time	Finnish Date & Time	Name	Signature

	Care Home Cleaning Tasks - Communal Area	M	T	W	T	F	S	S	Cleaned By	Checked By	Date/Tim
1	Clean And Sanitize All The Desks And Tables										
2	Clean And Sanitize All The Counter Tops And Surface Areas										
3	Wipe Down The Walls Wherever There Are Spills And Splashes										
4	Disinfect Touch Points, Light Switches And Other Switches										
5	Clean And Disinfect All Doors, Handles And Doorknobs										
6	Clean And Dust Door Frames, Remember To Dust The Tops										
7	Dust Light Fixtures & Shades With A Duster Or A Microfibre Cloth										
8	Clean And Wipe Mirrors Remove Fingerprints, Smears & Dirt										
9	Clean And Sanitize Over Chair Tables										
10	Clean And Polish Bookshelves, Remember To Dust The Top										
11	Remove, Wash And Clean Any Dirty Cups Or Glasses										
12	Remove, Wash And Clean Any Dirty Plates, Bowels Or Cutlery										
13	Clean And Sanitize Any Chairs, Seats And Benches										
14	Water Jugs (Washed Thoroughly Each Day & Re-Filled)										
15	Water Any Plants And Flowers										
16	Dust Plant Leafs (A Healthy Plant Needs To Be Clear Of Dust)										
17	Empty The Waste Baskets And Recycling Bins										
18	Clean And Disinfectant The Waste Bins And Recycling Bins										
19	Clean And Wipe Down Windowsills										
20	Spray Air Freshener This Keeps The Room Smelling Fresh										
21	Clean And Disinfect Cabinets And Units										
22	Clean And Sanitize Desk Accessories										
23	Replace Dirty Table Linen And Move To Laundry Room										
24	Polish Any Wooden Furniture And Hardwood Surfaces										
25	Clean Skirting Boards/Baseboards And Corners										
26	Clean And Polish Fireplace Mantelpiece And Surrounds										
27	Wipe Down Equipment & Sanitize Tea And Coffee Making Facilities										
28	Clean And Sanitize Telephones, Cords/Leads & All Touch Points										
29	Clean And Sanitize Walking Sticks And Any Other Walking Aids										

Care Home Cleaning Tasks - Communal Area	M	T	W	T	F	S	S	Cleaned By	Checked By	Date/Time
Dust Television, Top Sides And Back, TV Unit And TV Stand										
Clean TV Screen With Soft Damp Cloth (Use Water/Cleaner)										
Vacuum/Hoover Between Furniture And The Walls										
Clean And Sanitize All Wheelchairs										
Check For Broken Wheelchairs, Frames and Wheels										
Vacuum Under Furniture, Units, Tables And Cabinets										
Vacuum And Hoover The Carpets, Mats And Rugs										
Vacuum Furnishings, Cushions, Chairs, Sofas And Couches										
Steam Clean Carpets And Rugs										
Dust And Clean Any Picture Frames And Wall Art										
Clean & Check Contents Of Medicine Trolleys & Cupboards										
Clean & Vacuum The Desk Chair, Legs And Chair Wheels										
Wash And Clean Air Vents										
Dust Ceiling Fan Blades With Duster Or A Microfibre Cloth										
Wash And Clean Windows (Inside And Outside)										
Dust And Clean The Walls From Top To Bottom										
Clean Blinds (Dust The Blinds With A Damp Microfibre Cloth)										
Clean Curtains (Vacuum On A Low Setting Or Wash If Possible)										
Dust And Wash Radiator Covers										
Wash And Clean Ceiling Light Covers										
Clean & Vacuum Central Heating Units (Backs Of Radiators)										
Clean And Disinfect Any Handrails										
Clean And Sanitize Computer, Keyboard And Computer Mice										
Clean And Sanitize iPads, Tablets, Laptops & Mobile Phones										
Floors Mopped Clean With Cleaning Or Disinfecting Solution										
The Floors Are Swept And Free From Debris And Litter										
Clean Sliding Doors and Room Partitions										
Throw Away Outdated Newspapers, Magazines, Papers										
Check For Broken Furniture (Report/Schedule Maintenance)										
Light Bulbs Checked And None Functioning Bulbs Replaced										
Check Hardware, Door Stops And Lock Mechanisms										
Fire Exit Lights And Emergency Lights Checked & Functioning										
Test Carbon Monoxide Alarm And Replace Batteries If Required										
Test Smoke Detector Alarm And Replace Batteries If Required										
Paper Dispensers And Paper Towel Rolls Re-Stocked										
Soap Dispensers, Hand Sanitizers And Hand Gels Are Refilled										
Face Masks, Protective Gloves And Face Shields Re-Stocked										

CARE HOME TOILET & RESTROOM CLEANING *Checklist*

Building	Location	Room Number	Area

Start Date & Time	Finnish Date & Time	Name	Signature

	Care Home Cleaning Tasks - Toilet & Restroom	M	T	W	T	F	S	S	Cleaned By	Checked By	Date/Time
1	Clean And Sanitize All The Counter Tops And Surface Areas										
2	Wipe Down The Walls Wherever There Are Spills And Splashes										
3	Disinfect Touch Points, Light Switches And Other Switches										
4	Clean And Disinfect All Doors, Handles And Doorknobs										
5	Clean And Dust Door Frames, Remember To Dust The Tops										
6	Dust Light Fixtures With A Duster Or A Microfibre Cloth										
7	Wall Mirrors Cleaned With Glass Cleaner										
8	Clean Any Bathroom Glasses And Cups										
9	Clean And Sanitize Any Chairs And Seats										
10	Empty The Waste Basket And Recycling Bin										
11	Clean And Disinfectant The Waste Bin And Recycling Bin										
12	Clean And Wipe Down Windowsills										
13	Spray Air Freshener This Keeps The Room Smelling Fresh										
14	Air/Odour Control Systems Are Filled And Operating Correctly										
15	Clean Skirting Boards/Baseboards And Corners										
16	Vacuum And Hoover Bath Mats, Shower Mats And Rugs										
17	Replace Bath Mats, Shower Mats And Rugs With Clean Ones										
18	Steam Clean Carpets And Rugs										
19	Hand Towels Replaced With Fresh Clean Ones										
20	Bath Towels Replaced With Fresh Clean Ones										
21	Face Towels Replaced With Fresh Clean Ones										
22	Electric Hand Dryers Cleaned, Disinfected & Operating Correctly										
23	Soap Dispensers, Sanitizers And Hand Gels Are Refilled										
24	Clean & Check Contents Of Medicine Trolleys & Cupboards										
25	Clean And Disinfect Any Handrails										
26	Sinks, Taps And Fixtures Cleaned And Disinfected										
27	Clean And Disinfect Cabinets And Units										
28	Feminine Hygiene Dispensers Re-Stocked										
29	Feminine Hygiene Bins/Containers Emptied And Cleared										

Care Home Cleaning Tasks - Toilet & Restroom	M	T	W	T	F	S	S	Cleaned By	Checked By	Date/Time
Clean & Vacuum Central Heating Units (Backs Of Radiators)										
Wash And Clean Ceiling Light Covers										
Toilet Roll Holders And Toilet Rolls Re-Stocked										
Toilet Roll Holders Cleaned And Disinfected										
Clean Inside The Toilets And Urinals With Disinfectant										
Toilet Seats Cleaned And Disinfected										
Clean Top Of Toilets Tanks, The Bases And Behind Toilets										
Urinal Handles Cleaned And Disinfected										
Urinal Screens Cleaned, Disinfected And Blocks Replaced										
Paper Dispensers And Paper Towel Rolls Re-Stocked										
Paper Dispensers And Paper Towel Roll Cleaned & Disinfected										
The Floors Are Swept And Free From Debris And Litter										
Floors Mopped Clean With Cleaning Or Disinfecting Solution										
Put Up Or Place Wet Floor Signs After Mopping Floors										
Showers And Shower Heads, Cleaned And Disinfected										
Soak Shower Heads										
Clean And Disinfect Glass Shower Doors/Outer Doors										
Clean Soap Scum From Shower Walls										
Clean Blinds (Dust The Blinds With A Damp Microfibre Cloth)										
Clean Curtains (Vacuum On A Low Setting Or Wash If Possible)										
Dust And Wash Radiator Covers										
Clean And Disinfect Commodes Between Each Use										
Clean And Disinfect Shower Chairs Between Each Use										
Bath Hoists Cleaned And Disinfected Between Each Use										
Scrub Tub/Bath, Polish Facets And Taps, Clean & Disinfected										
Toothbrush Holders And Soap Holders Cleaned										
Re-Place Shower Curtains With Clean Fresh Ones										
Wash And Clean Air Vents										
Thoroughly Clean Grout And Tiles										
Disinfect And Clean All The Walls From Top To Bottom										
Wash And Clean Windows (Inside And Outside)										
Unclog The Drains (Sink, Bath And Shower)										
Pour Drain Cleaner Down Sink, Shower & Bath Drains										
Floor Drains And Drain Covers Are Open And Free Of Debris										
Hair Dryers Cleaned And Disinfected And Operating Correctly										
Light Bulbs Checked And None Functioning Bulbs Replaced										
Check Hardware, Door Stops And Lock Mechanisms										

CARE HOME BEDROOM CLEANING *Checklist*

Building	Location	Room Number	Area

Start Date & Time	Finnish Date & Time	Name	Signature

	Care Home Cleaning Tasks - Bedrooms	M	T	W	T	F	S	S	Cleaned By	Checked By	Date/Time
1	Clean And Sanitize All The Desks And Tables										
2	Clean And Sanitize All The Counter Tops And Surface Areas										
3	Wipe Down The Walls Wherever There Are Spills And Splashes										
4	Disinfect Touch Points, Light Switches And Other Switches										
5	Clean And Disinfect All Doors, Handles And Doorknobs										
6	Clean And Dust Door Frames, Remember To Dust The Tops										
7	Dust Light Fixtures With A Duster Or A Microfibre Cloth										
8	Clean & Wipe Mirrors Remove Fingerprints, Smears & Dirt										
9	Clean And Dust Bedside Cabinets										
10	Clean And Sanitize Over Chair Tables										
11	Clean And Sanitize Over Bed Tables										
12	Clean And Check Bed Frames										
13	Mattresses Hoovered And Cleaned With Disinfectant										
14	Clean And Polish Bookshelves, Remember To Dust The Top										
15	Remove, Wash And Clean Any Dirty Cups Or Glasses										
16	Remove, Wash And Clean Any Dirty Plates, Bowels Or Cutlery										
17	Clean And Sanitize Any Chairs And Seats										
18	Water Jug (Washed Thoroughly Each Day & Re-Filled)										
19	Water Any Plants And Flowers										
20	Dust Plant Leafs (A Healthy Plant Needs To Be Clear Of Dust)										
21	Empty The Waste Basket And Recycling Bin										
22	Clean And Disinfectant The Waste Bin And Recycling Bin										
23	Clean And Wipe Down Windowsills										
24	Spray Air Freshener This Keeps The Room Smelling Fresh										
25	Clean And Disinfect Cabinets And Units										
26	Clean And Sanitize Desk Accessories										
27	Replace Dirty Linen And Move To Laundry Room										
28	Polish Any Wooden Furniture And Hardwood Surfaces										
29	Clean Skirting Boards/Baseboards And Corners										

Care Home Cleaning Tasks - Bedrooms Continued	M	T	W	T	F	S	S	Cleaned By	Checked By	Date/Time
Dust Television, Top Sides And Back, TV Unit And TV Stand										
Clean TV Screen With Soft Damp Cloth (Use Water/Cleaner)										
Vacuum/Hoover Between Bedroom Furniture And The Walls										
Clean And Sanitize Resident's Personal Wheelchair										
Check For Broken Wheelchairs, Frames and Wheels										
Vacuum Under Furniture, Beds, Sofas and Dressers										
Vacuum And Hoover The Carpets, Mats And Rugs										
Vacuum Furnishings, Cushions, Chairs, Sofas And Couches										
Steam Clean Carpets And Rugs										
Dust And Clean Any Picture Frames And Photo Frames										
Ledges, Flat Surfaces And The Tops Of Wardrobes Dusted										
Clean & Check Contents Of Medicine Trolleys & Cupboards										
Clean And Sanitize Mobile Phone, Phone Case And Screen										
Clean & Vacuum The Desk Chair, Legs And Chair Wheels										
Wash And Clean Air Vents										
Dust Ceiling Fan Blades With Duster Or A Microfibre Cloth										
Wash And Clean Windows (Inside And Outside)										
Dust And Clean The Walls From Top To Bottom										
Clean Blinds (Dust The Blinds With A Damp Microfibre Cloth)										
Clean Curtains (Vacuum On A Low Setting Or Wash If Possible)										
Dust And Wash Radiator Covers										
Wash And Clean Ceiling Light Covers										
Clean & Vacuum Central Heating Units (Backs Of Radiators)										
Clean And Disinfect Any Handrails										
Hand Towels Replaced With Fresh Clean Ones										
Sink Wall Mirror Cleaned With Glass Cleaner										
Sinks, Taps And Fixtures Cleaned And Disinfected										
Pour Drain Cleaner Down Sink Drains										
Check For Broken Furniture (Report/Schedule Maintenance)										
Light Bulbs Checked And None Functioning Bulbs Replaced										
Check Hardware, Door Stops And Lock Mechanisms										
Fire Exit Lights And Emergency Lights Checked & Functioning										
Test Carbon Monoxide Alarm And Replace Batteries If Required										
Test Smoke Detector Alarm And Replace Batteries If Required										
Paper Dispensers And Paper Towel Rolls Re-Stocked										
Soap Dispensers, Hand Sanitizers And Hand Gels Are Refilled										
Face Masks, Protective Gloves And Face Shields Re-Stocked										

CARE HOME COMMUNAL AREA CLEANING *Checklist*

Building	Location	Room Number	Area

Start Date & Time	Finnish Date & Time	Name	Signature

	Care Home Cleaning Tasks - Communal Area	M	T	W	T	F	S	S	Cleaned By	Checked By	Date/Tim
1	Clean And Sanitize All The Desks And Tables										
2	Clean And Sanitize All The Counter Tops And Surface Areas										
3	Wipe Down The Walls Wherever There Are Spills And Splashes										
4	Disinfect Touch Points, Light Switches And Other Switches										
5	Clean And Disinfect All Doors, Handles And Doorknobs										
6	Clean And Dust Door Frames, Remember To Dust The Tops										
7	Dust Light Fixtures & Shades With A Duster Or A Microfibre Cloth										
8	Clean And Wipe Mirrors Remove Fingerprints, Smears & Dirt										
9	Clean And Sanitize Over Chair Tables										
10	Clean And Polish Bookshelves, Remember To Dust The Top										
11	Remove, Wash And Clean Any Dirty Cups Or Glasses										
12	Remove, Wash And Clean Any Dirty Plates, Bowels Or Cutlery										
13	Clean And Sanitize Any Chairs, Seats And Benches										
14	Water Jugs (Washed Thoroughly Each Day & Re-Filled)										
15	Water Any Plants And Flowers										
16	Dust Plant Leafs (A Healthy Plant Needs To Be Clear Of Dust)										
17	Empty The Waste Baskets And Recycling Bins										
18	Clean And Disinfectant The Waste Bins And Recycling Bins										
19	Clean And Wipe Down Windowsills										
20	Spray Air Freshener This Keeps The Room Smelling Fresh										
21	Clean And Disinfect Cabinets And Units										
22	Clean And Sanitize Desk Accessories										
23	Replace Dirty Table Linen And Move To Laundry Room										
24	Polish Any Wooden Furniture And Hardwood Surfaces										
25	Clean Skirting Boards/Baseboards And Corners										
26	Clean And Polish Fireplace Mantelpiece And Surrounds										
27	Wipe Down Equipment & Sanitize Tea And Coffee Making Facilities										
28	Clean And Sanitize Telephones, Cords/Leads & All Touch Points										
29	Clean And Sanitize Walking Sticks And Any Other Walking Aids										

Care Home Cleaning Tasks - Communal Area	M	T	W	T	F	S	S	Cleaned By	Checked By	Date/Time
Dust Television, Top Sides And Back, TV Unit And TV Stand										
Clean TV Screen With Soft Damp Cloth (Use Water/Cleaner)										
Vacuum/Hoover Between Furniture And The Walls										
Clean And Sanitize All Wheelchairs										
Check For Broken Wheelchairs, Frames and Wheels										
Vacuum Under Furniture, Units, Tables And Cabinets										
Vacuum And Hoover The Carpets, Mats And Rugs										
Vacuum Furnishings, Cushions, Chairs, Sofas And Couches										
Steam Clean Carpets And Rugs										
Dust And Clean Any Picture Frames And Wall Art										
Clean & Check Contents Of Medicine Trolleys & Cupboards										
Clean & Vacuum The Desk Chair, Legs And Chair Wheels										
Wash And Clean Air Vents										
Dust Ceiling Fan Blades With Duster Or A Microfibre Cloth										
Wash And Clean Windows (Inside And Outside)										
Dust And Clean The Walls From Top To Bottom										
Clean Blinds (Dust The Blinds With A Damp Microfibre Cloth)										
Clean Curtains (Vacuum On A Low Setting Or Wash If Possible)										
Dust And Wash Radiator Covers										
Wash And Clean Ceiling Light Covers										
Clean & Vacuum Central Heating Units (Backs Of Radiators)										
Clean And Disinfect Any Handrails										
Clean And Sanitize Computer, Keyboard And Computer Mice										
Clean And Sanitize iPads, Tablets, Laptops & Mobile Phones										
Floors Mopped Clean With Cleaning Or Disinfecting Solution										
The Floors Are Swept And Free From Debris And Litter										
Clean Sliding Doors and Room Partitions										
Throw Away Outdated Newspapers, Magazines, Papers										
Check For Broken Furniture (Report/Schedule Maintenance)										
Light Bulbs Checked And None Functioning Bulbs Replaced										
Check Hardware, Door Stops And Lock Mechanisms										
Fire Exit Lights And Emergency Lights Checked & Functioning										
Test Carbon Monoxide Alarm And Replace Batteries If Required										
Test Smoke Detector Alarm And Replace Batteries If Required										
Paper Dispensers And Paper Towel Rolls Re-Stocked										
Soap Dispensers, Hand Sanitizers And Hand Gels Are Refilled										
Face Masks, Protective Gloves And Face Shields Re-Stocked										

CARE HOME TOILET & RESTROOM CLEANING *Checklist*

Building	Location	Room Number	Area

Start Date & Time	Finnish Date & Time	Name	Signature

	Care Home Cleaning Tasks - Toilet & Restroom	M	T	W	T	F	S	S	Cleaned By	Checked By	Date/Time
1	Clean And Sanitize All The Counter Tops And Surface Areas										
2	Wipe Down The Walls Wherever There Are Spills And Splashes										
3	Disinfect Touch Points, Light Switches And Other Switches										
4	Clean And Disinfect All Doors, Handles And Doorknobs										
5	Clean And Dust Door Frames, Remember To Dust The Tops										
6	Dust Light Fixtures With A Duster Or A Microfibre Cloth										
7	Wall Mirrors Cleaned With Glass Cleaner										
8	Clean Any Bathroom Glasses And Cups										
9	Clean And Sanitize Any Chairs And Seats										
10	Empty The Waste Basket And Recycling Bin										
11	Clean And Disinfectant The Waste Bin And Recycling Bin										
12	Clean And Wipe Down Windowsills										
13	Spray Air Freshener This Keeps The Room Smelling Fresh										
14	Air/Odour Control Systems Are Filled And Operating Correctly										
15	Clean Skirting Boards/Baseboards And Corners										
16	Vacuum And Hoover Bath Mats, Shower Mats And Rugs										
17	Replace Bath Mats, Shower Mats And Rugs With Clean Ones										
18	Steam Clean Carpets And Rugs										
19	Hand Towels Replaced With Fresh Clean Ones										
20	Bath Towels Replaced With Fresh Clean Ones										
21	Face Towels Replaced With Fresh Clean Ones										
22	Electric Hand Dryers Cleaned, Disinfected & Operating Correctly										
23	Soap Dispensers, Sanitizers And Hand Gels Are Refilled										
24	Clean & Check Contents Of Medicine Trolleys & Cupboards										
25	Clean And Disinfect Any Handrails										
26	Sinks, Taps And Fixtures Cleaned And Disinfected										
27	Clean And Disinfect Cabinets And Units										
28	Feminine Hygiene Dispensers Re-Stocked										
29	Feminine Hygiene Bins/Containers Emptied And Cleared										

Care Home Cleaning Tasks - Toilet & Restroom	M	T	W	T	F	S	S	Cleaned By	Checked By	Date/Time
Clean & Vacuum Central Heating Units (Backs Of Radiators)										
Wash And Clean Ceiling Light Covers										
Toilet Roll Holders And Toilet Rolls Re-Stocked										
Toilet Roll Holders Cleaned And Disinfected										
Clean Inside The Toilets And Urinals With Disinfectant										
Toilet Seats Cleaned And Disinfected										
Clean Top Of Toilets Tanks, The Bases And Behind Toilets										
Urinal Handles Cleaned And Disinfected										
Urinal Screens Cleaned, Disinfected And Blocks Replaced										
Paper Dispensers And Paper Towel Rolls Re-Stocked										
Paper Dispensers And Paper Towel Roll Cleaned & Disinfected										
The Floors Are Swept And Free From Debris And Litter										
Floors Mopped Clean With Cleaning Or Disinfecting Solution										
Put Up Or Place Wet Floor Signs After Mopping Floors										
Showers And Shower Heads, Cleaned And Disinfected										
Soak Shower Heads										
Clean And Disinfect Glass Shower Doors/Outer Doors										
Clean Soap Scum From Shower Walls										
Clean Blinds (Dust The Blinds With A Damp Microfibre Cloth)										
Clean Curtains (Vacuum On A Low Setting Or Wash If Possible)										
Dust And Wash Radiator Covers										
Clean And Disinfect Commodes Between Each Use										
Clean And Disinfect Shower Chairs Between Each Use										
Bath Hoists Cleaned And Disinfected Between Each Use										
Scrub Tub/Bath, Polish Facets And Taps, Clean & Disinfected										
Toothbrush Holders And Soap Holders Cleaned										
Re-Place Shower Curtains With Clean Fresh Ones										
Wash And Clean Air Vents										
Thoroughly Clean Grout And Tiles										
Disinfect And Clean All The Walls From Top To Bottom										
Wash And Clean Windows (Inside And Outside)										
Unclog The Drains (Sink, Bath And Shower)										
Pour Drain Cleaner Down Sink, Shower & Bath Drains										
Floor Drains And Drain Covers Are Open And Free Of Debris										
Hair Dryers Cleaned And Disinfected And Operating Correctly										
Light Bulbs Checked And None Functioning Bulbs Replaced										
Check Hardware, Door Stops And Lock Mechanisms										

CARE HOME BEDROOM CLEANING *Checklist*

Building	Location	Room Number	Area

Start Date & Time	Finnish Date & Time	Name	Signature

	Care Home Cleaning Tasks - Bedrooms	M	T	W	T	F	S	S	Cleaned By	Checked By	Date/Tim
1	Clean And Sanitize All The Desks And Tables										
2	Clean And Sanitize All The Counter Tops And Surface Areas										
3	Wipe Down The Walls Wherever There Are Spills And Splashes										
4	Disinfect Touch Points, Light Switches And Other Switches										
5	Clean And Disinfect All Doors, Handles And Doorknobs										
6	Clean And Dust Door Frames, Remember To Dust The Tops										
7	Dust Light Fixtures With A Duster Or A Microfibre Cloth										
8	Clean & Wipe Mirrors Remove Fingerprints, Smears & Dirt										
9	Clean And Dust Bedside Cabinets										
10	Clean And Sanitize Over Chair Tables										
11	Clean And Sanitize Over Bed Tables										
12	Clean And Check Bed Frames										
13	Mattresses Hoovered And Cleaned With Disinfectant										
14	Clean And Polish Bookshelves, Remember To Dust The Top										
15	Remove, Wash And Clean Any Dirty Cups Or Glasses										
16	Remove, Wash And Clean Any Dirty Plates, Bowels Or Cutlery										
17	Clean And Sanitize Any Chairs And Seats										
18	Water Jug (Washed Thoroughly Each Day & Re-Filled)										
19	Water Any Plants And Flowers										
20	Dust Plant Leafs (A Healthy Plant Needs To Be Clear Of Dust)										
21	Empty The Waste Basket And Recycling Bin										
22	Clean And Disinfectant The Waste Bin And Recycling Bin										
23	Clean And Wipe Down Windowsills										
24	Spray Air Freshener This Keeps The Room Smelling Fresh										
25	Clean And Disinfect Cabinets And Units										
26	Clean And Sanitize Desk Accessories										
27	Replace Dirty Linen And Move To Laundry Room										
28	Polish Any Wooden Furniture And Hardwood Surfaces										
29	Clean Skirting Boards/Baseboards And Corners										

Care Home Cleaning Tasks - Bedrooms Continued	M	T	W	T	F	S	S	Cleaned By	Checked By	Date/Time
Dust Television, Top Sides And Back, TV Unit And TV Stand										
Clean TV Screen With Soft Damp Cloth (Use Water/Cleaner)										
Vacuum/Hoover Between Bedroom Furniture And The Walls										
Clean And Sanitize Resident's Personal Wheelchair										
Check For Broken Wheelchairs, Frames and Wheels										
Vacuum Under Furniture, Beds, Sofas and Dressers										
Vacuum And Hoover The Carpets, Mats And Rugs										
Vacuum Furnishings, Cushions, Chairs, Sofas And Couches										
Steam Clean Carpets And Rugs										
Dust And Clean Any Picture Frames And Photo Frames										
Ledges, Flat Surfaces And The Tops Of Wardrobes Dusted										
Clean & Check Contents Of Medicine Trolleys & Cupboards										
Clean And Sanitize Mobile Phone, Phone Case And Screen										
Clean & Vacuum The Desk Chair, Legs And Chair Wheels										
Wash And Clean Air Vents										
Dust Ceiling Fan Blades With Duster Or A Microfibre Cloth										
Wash And Clean Windows (Inside And Outside)										
Dust And Clean The Walls From Top To Bottom										
Clean Blinds (Dust The Blinds With A Damp Microfibre Cloth)										
Clean Curtains (Vacuum On A Low Setting Or Wash If Possible)										
Dust And Wash Radiator Covers										
Wash And Clean Ceiling Light Covers										
Clean & Vacuum Central Heating Units (Backs Of Radiators)										
Clean And Disinfect Any Handrails										
Hand Towels Replaced With Fresh Clean Ones										
Sink Wall Mirror Cleaned With Glass Cleaner										
Sinks, Taps And Fixtures Cleaned And Disinfected										
Pour Drain Cleaner Down Sink Drains										
Check For Broken Furniture (Report/Schedule Maintenance)										
Light Bulbs Checked And None Functioning Bulbs Replaced										
Check Hardware, Door Stops And Lock Mechanisms										
Fire Exit Lights And Emergency Lights Checked & Functioning										
Test Carbon Monoxide Alarm And Replace Batteries If Required										
Test Smoke Detector Alarm And Replace Batteries If Required										
Paper Dispensers And Paper Towel Rolls Re-Stocked										
Soap Dispensers, Hand Sanitizers And Hand Gels Are Refilled										
Face Masks, Protective Gloves And Face Shields Re-Stocked										

CARE HOME COMMUNAL AREA CLEANING *Checklist*

Building	Location	Room Number	Area

Start Date & Time	Finnish Date & Time	Name	Signature

	Care Home Cleaning Tasks - Communal Area	M	T	W	T	F	S	S	Cleaned By	Checked By	Date/Time
1	Clean And Sanitize All The Desks And Tables										
2	Clean And Sanitize All The Counter Tops And Surface Areas										
3	Wipe Down The Walls Wherever There Are Spills And Splashes										
4	Disinfect Touch Points, Light Switches And Other Switches										
5	Clean And Disinfect All Doors, Handles And Doorknobs										
6	Clean And Dust Door Frames, Remember To Dust The Tops										
7	Dust Light Fixtures & Shades With A Duster Or A Microfibre Cloth										
8	Clean And Wipe Mirrors Remove Fingerprints, Smears & Dirt										
9	Clean And Sanitize Over Chair Tables										
10	Clean And Polish Bookshelves, Remember To Dust The Top										
11	Remove, Wash And Clean Any Dirty Cups Or Glasses										
12	Remove, Wash And Clean Any Dirty Plates, Bowels Or Cutlery										
13	Clean And Sanitize Any Chairs, Seats And Benches										
14	Water Jugs (Washed Thoroughly Each Day & Re-Filled)										
15	Water Any Plants And Flowers										
16	Dust Plant Leafs (A Healthy Plant Needs To Be Clear Of Dust)										
17	Empty The Waste Baskets And Recycling Bins										
18	Clean And Disinfectant The Waste Bins And Recycling Bins										
19	Clean And Wipe Down Windowsills										
20	Spray Air Freshener This Keeps The Room Smelling Fresh										
21	Clean And Disinfect Cabinets And Units										
22	Clean And Sanitize Desk Accessories										
23	Replace Dirty Table Linen And Move To Laundry Room										
24	Polish Any Wooden Furniture And Hardwood Surfaces										
25	Clean Skirting Boards/Baseboards And Corners										
26	Clean And Polish Fireplace Mantelpiece And Surrounds										
27	Wipe Down Equipment & Sanitize Tea And Coffee Making Facilities										
28	Clean And Sanitize Telephones, Cords/Leads & All Touch Points										
29	Clean And Sanitize Walking Sticks And Any Other Walking Aids										

Care Home Cleaning Tasks - Communal Area	M	T	W	T	F	S	S	Cleaned By	Checked By	Date/Time
Dust Television, Top Sides And Back, TV Unit And TV Stand										
Clean TV Screen With Soft Damp Cloth (Use Water/Cleaner)										
Vacuum/Hoover Between Furniture And The Walls										
Clean And Sanitize All Wheelchairs										
Check For Broken Wheelchairs, Frames and Wheels										
Vacuum Under Furniture, Units, Tables And Cabinets										
Vacuum And Hoover The Carpets, Mats And Rugs										
Vacuum Furnishings, Cushions, Chairs, Sofas And Couches										
Steam Clean Carpets And Rugs										
Dust And Clean Any Picture Frames And Wall Art										
Clean & Check Contents Of Medicine Trolleys & Cupboards										
Clean & Vacuum The Desk Chair, Legs And Chair Wheels										
Wash And Clean Air Vents										
Dust Ceiling Fan Blades With Duster Or A Microfibre Cloth										
Wash And Clean Windows (Inside And Outside)										
Dust And Clean The Walls From Top To Bottom										
Clean Blinds (Dust The Blinds With A Damp Microfibre Cloth)										
Clean Curtains (Vacuum On A Low Setting Or Wash If Possible)										
Dust And Wash Radiator Covers										
Wash And Clean Ceiling Light Covers										
Clean & Vacuum Central Heating Units (Backs Of Radiators)										
Clean And Disinfect Any Handrails										
Clean And Sanitize Computer, Keyboard And Computer Mice										
Clean And Sanitize iPads, Tablets, Laptops & Mobile Phones										
Floors Mopped Clean With Cleaning Or Disinfecting Solution										
The Floors Are Swept And Free From Debris And Litter										
Clean Sliding Doors and Room Partitions										
Throw Away Outdated Newspapers, Magazines, Papers										
Check For Broken Furniture (Report/Schedule Maintenance)										
Light Bulbs Checked And None Functioning Bulbs Replaced										
Check Hardware, Door Stops And Lock Mechanisms										
Fire Exit Lights And Emergency Lights Checked & Functioning										
Test Carbon Monoxide Alarm And Replace Batteries If Required										
Test Smoke Detector Alarm And Replace Batteries If Required										
Paper Dispensers And Paper Towel Rolls Re-Stocked										
Soap Dispensers, Hand Sanitizers And Hand Gels Are Refilled										
Face Masks, Protective Gloves And Face Shields Re-Stocked										

CARE HOME TOILET & RESTROOM CLEANING *Checklist*

Building	Location	Room Number	Area

Start Date & Time	Finnish Date & Time	Name	Signature

	Care Home Cleaning Tasks - Toilet & Restroom	M	T	W	T	F	S	S	Cleaned By	Checked By	Date/Tim
1	Clean And Sanitize All The Counter Tops And Surface Areas										
2	Wipe Down The Walls Wherever There Are Spills And Splashes										
3	Disinfect Touch Points, Light Switches And Other Switches										
4	Clean And Disinfect All Doors, Handles And Doorknobs										
5	Clean And Dust Door Frames, Remember To Dust The Tops										
6	Dust Light Fixtures With A Duster Or A Microfibre Cloth										
7	Wall Mirrors Cleaned With Glass Cleaner										
8	Clean Any Bathroom Glasses And Cups										
9	Clean And Sanitize Any Chairs And Seats										
10	Empty The Waste Basket And Recycling Bin										
11	Clean And Disinfectant The Waste Bin And Recycling Bin										
12	Clean And Wipe Down Windowsills										
13	Spray Air Freshener This Keeps The Room Smelling Fresh										
14	Air/Odour Control Systems Are Filled And Operating Correctly										
15	Clean Skirting Boards/Baseboards And Corners										
16	Vacuum And Hoover Bath Mats, Shower Mats And Rugs										
17	Replace Bath Mats, Shower Mats And Rugs With Clean Ones										
18	Steam Clean Carpets And Rugs										
19	Hand Towels Replaced With Fresh Clean Ones										
20	Bath Towels Replaced With Fresh Clean Ones										
21	Face Towels Replaced With Fresh Clean Ones										
22	Electric Hand Dryers Cleaned, Disinfected & Operating Correctly										
23	Soap Dispensers, Sanitizers And Hand Gels Are Refilled										
24	Clean & Check Contents Of Medicine Trolleys & Cupboards										
25	Clean And Disinfect Any Handrails										
26	Sinks, Taps And Fixtures Cleaned And Disinfected										
27	Clean And Disinfect Cabinets And Units										
28	Feminine Hygiene Dispensers Re-Stocked										
29	Feminine Hygiene Bins/Containers Emptied And Cleared										

Care Home Cleaning Tasks - Toilet & Restroom	M	T	W	T	F	S	S	Cleaned By	Checked By	Date/Time
Clean & Vacuum Central Heating Units (Backs Of Radiators)										
Wash And Clean Ceiling Light Covers										
Toilet Roll Holders And Toilet Rolls Re-Stocked										
Toilet Roll Holders Cleaned And Disinfected										
Clean Inside The Toilets And Urinals With Disinfectant										
Toilet Seats Cleaned And Disinfected										
Clean Top Of Toilets Tanks, The Bases And Behind Toilets										
Urinal Handles Cleaned And Disinfected										
Urinal Screens Cleaned, Disinfected And Blocks Replaced										
Paper Dispensers And Paper Towel Rolls Re-Stocked										
Paper Dispensers And Paper Towel Roll Cleaned & Disinfected										
The Floors Are Swept And Free From Debris And Litter										
Floors Mopped Clean With Cleaning Or Disinfecting Solution										
Put Up Or Place Wet Floor Signs After Mopping Floors										
Showers And Shower Heads, Cleaned And Disinfected										
Soak Shower Heads										
Clean And Disinfect Glass Shower Doors/Outer Doors										
Clean Soap Scum From Shower Walls										
Clean Blinds (Dust The Blinds With A Damp Microfibre Cloth)										
Clean Curtains (Vacuum On A Low Setting Or Wash If Possible)										
Dust And Wash Radiator Covers										
Clean And Disinfect Commodes Between Each Use										
Clean And Disinfect Shower Chairs Between Each Use										
Bath Hoists Cleaned And Disinfected Between Each Use										
Scrub Tub/Bath, Polish Facets And Taps, Clean & Disinfected										
Toothbrush Holders And Soap Holders Cleaned										
Re-Place Shower Curtains With Clean Fresh Ones										
Wash And Clean Air Vents										
Thoroughly Clean Grout And Tiles										
Disinfect And Clean All The Walls From Top To Bottom										
Wash And Clean Windows (Inside And Outside)										
Unclog The Drains (Sink, Bath And Shower)										
Pour Drain Cleaner Down Sink, Shower & Bath Drains										
Floor Drains And Drain Covers Are Open And Free Of Debris										
Hair Dryers Cleaned And Disinfected And Operating Correctly										
Light Bulbs Checked And None Functioning Bulbs Replaced										
Check Hardware, Door Stops And Lock Mechanisms										

CARE HOME BEDROOM CLEANING *Checklist*

Building	Location	Room Number	Area

Start Date & Time	Finnish Date & Time	Name	Signature

	Care Home Cleaning Tasks - Bedrooms	M	T	W	T	F	S	S	Cleaned By	Checked By	Date/Time
1	Clean And Sanitize All The Desks And Tables										
2	Clean And Sanitize All The Counter Tops And Surface Areas										
3	Wipe Down The Walls Wherever There Are Spills And Splashes										
4	Disinfect Touch Points, Light Switches And Other Switches										
5	Clean And Disinfect All Doors, Handles And Doorknobs										
6	Clean And Dust Door Frames, Remember To Dust The Tops										
7	Dust Light Fixtures With A Duster Or A Microfibre Cloth										
8	Clean & Wipe Mirrors Remove Fingerprints, Smears & Dirt										
9	Clean And Dust Bedside Cabinets										
10	Clean And Sanitize Over Chair Tables										
11	Clean And Sanitize Over Bed Tables										
12	Clean And Check Bed Frames										
13	Mattresses Hoovered And Cleaned With Disinfectant										
14	Clean And Polish Bookshelves, Remember To Dust The Top										
15	Remove, Wash And Clean Any Dirty Cups Or Glasses										
16	Remove, Wash And Clean Any Dirty Plates, Bowels Or Cutlery										
17	Clean And Sanitize Any Chairs And Seats										
18	Water Jug (Washed Thoroughly Each Day & Re-Filled)										
19	Water Any Plants And Flowers										
20	Dust Plant Leafs (A Healthy Plant Needs To Be Clear Of Dust)										
21	Empty The Waste Basket And Recycling Bin										
22	Clean And Disinfectant The Waste Bin And Recycling Bin										
23	Clean And Wipe Down Windowsills										
24	Spray Air Freshener This Keeps The Room Smelling Fresh										
25	Clean And Disinfect Cabinets And Units										
26	Clean And Sanitize Desk Accessories										
27	Replace Dirty Linen And Move To Laundry Room										
28	Polish Any Wooden Furniture And Hardwood Surfaces										
29	Clean Skirting Boards/Baseboards And Corners										

Care Home Cleaning Tasks - Bedrooms Continued	M	T	W	T	F	S	S	Cleaned By	Checked By	Date/Time
Dust Television, Top Sides And Back, TV Unit And TV Stand										
Clean TV Screen With Soft Damp Cloth (Use Water/Cleaner)										
Vacuum/Hoover Between Bedroom Furniture And The Walls										
Clean And Sanitize Resident's Personal Wheelchair										
Check For Broken Wheelchairs, Frames and Wheels										
Vacuum Under Furniture, Beds, Sofas and Dressers										
Vacuum And Hoover The Carpets, Mats And Rugs										
Vacuum Furnishings, Cushions, Chairs, Sofas And Couches										
Steam Clean Carpets And Rugs										
Dust And Clean Any Picture Frames And Photo Frames										
Ledges, Flat Surfaces And The Tops Of Wardrobes Dusted										
Clean & Check Contents Of Medicine Trolleys & Cupboards										
Clean And Sanitize Mobile Phone, Phone Case And Screen										
Clean & Vacuum The Desk Chair, Legs And Chair Wheels										
Wash And Clean Air Vents										
Dust Ceiling Fan Blades With Duster Or A Microfibre Cloth										
Wash And Clean Windows (Inside And Outside)										
Dust And Clean The Walls From Top To Bottom										
Clean Blinds (Dust The Blinds With A Damp Microfibre Cloth)										
Clean Curtains (Vacuum On A Low Setting Or Wash If Possible)										
Dust And Wash Radiator Covers										
Wash And Clean Ceiling Light Covers										
Clean & Vacuum Central Heating Units (Backs Of Radiators)										
Clean And Disinfect Any Handrails										
Hand Towels Replaced With Fresh Clean Ones										
Sink Wall Mirror Cleaned With Glass Cleaner										
Sinks, Taps And Fixtures Cleaned And Disinfected										
Pour Drain Cleaner Down Sink Drains										
Check For Broken Furniture (Report/Schedule Maintenance)										
Light Bulbs Checked And None Functioning Bulbs Replaced										
Check Hardware, Door Stops And Lock Mechanisms										
Fire Exit Lights And Emergency Lights Checked & Functioning										
Test Carbon Monoxide Alarm And Replace Batteries If Required										
Test Smoke Detector Alarm And Replace Batteries If Required										
Paper Dispensers And Paper Towel Rolls Re-Stocked										
Soap Dispensers, Hand Sanitizers And Hand Gels Are Refilled										
Face Masks, Protective Gloves And Face Shields Re-Stocked										

CARE HOME COMMUNAL AREA CLEANING *Checklist*

Building	Location	Room Number	Area

Start Date & Time	Finnish Date & Time	Name	Signature

	Care Home Cleaning Tasks - Communal Area	M	T	W	T	F	S	S	Cleaned By	Checked By	Date/Time
1	Clean And Sanitize All The Desks And Tables										
2	Clean And Sanitize All The Counter Tops And Surface Areas										
3	Wipe Down The Walls Wherever There Are Spills And Splashes										
4	Disinfect Touch Points, Light Switches And Other Switches										
5	Clean And Disinfect All Doors, Handles And Doorknobs										
6	Clean And Dust Door Frames, Remember To Dust The Tops										
7	Dust Light Fixtures & Shades With A Duster Or A Microfibre Cloth										
8	Clean And Wipe Mirrors Remove Fingerprints, Smears & Dirt										
9	Clean And Sanitize Over Chair Tables										
10	Clean And Polish Bookshelves, Remember To Dust The Top										
11	Remove, Wash And Clean Any Dirty Cups Or Glasses										
12	Remove, Wash And Clean Any Dirty Plates, Bowels Or Cutlery										
13	Clean And Sanitize Any Chairs, Seats And Benches										
14	Water Jugs (Washed Thoroughly Each Day & Re-Filled)										
15	Water Any Plants And Flowers										
16	Dust Plant Leafs (A Healthy Plant Needs To Be Clear Of Dust)										
17	Empty The Waste Baskets And Recycling Bins										
18	Clean And Disinfectant The Waste Bins And Recycling Bins										
19	Clean And Wipe Down Windowsills										
20	Spray Air Freshener This Keeps The Room Smelling Fresh										
21	Clean And Disinfect Cabinets And Units										
22	Clean And Sanitize Desk Accessories										
23	Replace Dirty Table Linen And Move To Laundry Room										
24	Polish Any Wooden Furniture And Hardwood Surfaces										
25	Clean Skirting Boards/Baseboards And Corners										
26	Clean And Polish Fireplace Mantelpiece And Surrounds										
27	Wipe Down Equipment & Sanitize Tea And Coffee Making Facilities										
28	Clean And Sanitize Telephones, Cords/Leads & All Touch Points										
29	Clean And Sanitize Walking Sticks And Any Other Walking Aids										

Care Home Cleaning Tasks - Communal Area	M	T	W	T	F	S	S	Cleaned By	Checked By	Date/Time
Dust Television, Top Sides And Back, TV Unit And TV Stand										
Clean TV Screen With Soft Damp Cloth (Use Water/Cleaner)										
Vacuum/Hoover Between Furniture And The Walls										
Clean And Sanitize All Wheelchairs										
Check For Broken Wheelchairs, Frames and Wheels										
Vacuum Under Furniture, Units, Tables And Cabinets										
Vacuum And Hoover The Carpets, Mats And Rugs										
Vacuum Furnishings, Cushions, Chairs, Sofas And Couches										
Steam Clean Carpets And Rugs										
Dust And Clean Any Picture Frames And Wall Art										
Clean & Check Contents Of Medicine Trolleys & Cupboards										
Clean & Vacuum The Desk Chair, Legs And Chair Wheels										
Wash And Clean Air Vents										
Dust Ceiling Fan Blades With Duster Or A Microfibre Cloth										
Wash And Clean Windows (Inside And Outside)										
Dust And Clean The Walls From Top To Bottom										
Clean Blinds (Dust The Blinds With A Damp Microfibre Cloth)										
Clean Curtains (Vacuum On A Low Setting Or Wash If Possible)										
Dust And Wash Radiator Covers										
Wash And Clean Ceiling Light Covers										
Clean & Vacuum Central Heating Units (Backs Of Radiators)										
Clean And Disinfect Any Handrails										
Clean And Sanitize Computer, Keyboard And Computer Mice										
Clean And Sanitize iPads, Tablets, Laptops & Mobile Phones										
Floors Mopped Clean With Cleaning Or Disinfecting Solution										
The Floors Are Swept And Free From Debris And Litter										
Clean Sliding Doors and Room Partitions										
Throw Away Outdated Newspapers, Magazines, Papers										
Check For Broken Furniture (Report/Schedule Maintenance)										
Light Bulbs Checked And None Functioning Bulbs Replaced										
Check Hardware, Door Stops And Lock Mechanisms										
Fire Exit Lights And Emergency Lights Checked & Functioning										
Test Carbon Monoxide Alarm And Replace Batteries If Required										
Test Smoke Detector Alarm And Replace Batteries If Required										
Paper Dispensers And Paper Towel Rolls Re-Stocked										
Soap Dispensers, Hand Sanitizers And Hand Gels Are Refilled										
Face Masks, Protective Gloves And Face Shields Re-Stocked										

CARE HOME TOILET & RESTROOM CLEANING *Checklis*

Building	Location	Room Number	Area

Start Date & Time	Finnish Date & Time	Name	Signature

	Care Home Cleaning Tasks - Toilet & Restroom	M	T	W	T	F	S	S	Cleaned By	Checked By	Date/Tim
1	Clean And Sanitize All The Counter Tops And Surface Areas										
2	Wipe Down The Walls Wherever There Are Spills And Splashes										
3	Disinfect Touch Points, Light Switches And Other Switches										
4	Clean And Disinfect All Doors, Handles And Doorknobs										
5	Clean And Dust Door Frames, Remember To Dust The Tops										
6	Dust Light Fixtures With A Duster Or A Microfibre Cloth										
7	Wall Mirrors Cleaned With Glass Cleaner										
8	Clean Any Bathroom Glasses And Cups										
9	Clean And Sanitize Any Chairs And Seats										
10	Empty The Waste Basket And Recycling Bin										
11	Clean And Disinfectant The Waste Bin And Recycling Bin										
12	Clean And Wipe Down Windowsills										
13	Spray Air Freshener This Keeps The Room Smelling Fresh										
14	Air/Odour Control Systems Are Filled And Operating Correctly										
15	Clean Skirting Boards/Baseboards And Corners										
16	Vacuum And Hoover Bath Mats, Shower Mats And Rugs										
17	Replace Bath Mats, Shower Mats And Rugs With Clean Ones										
18	Steam Clean Carpets And Rugs										
19	Hand Towels Replaced With Fresh Clean Ones										
20	Bath Towels Replaced With Fresh Clean Ones										
21	Face Towels Replaced With Fresh Clean Ones										
22	Electric Hand Dryers Cleaned, Disinfected & Operating Correctly										
23	Soap Dispensers, Sanitizers And Hand Gels Are Refilled										
24	Clean & Check Contents Of Medicine Trolleys & Cupboards										
25	Clean And Disinfect Any Handrails										
26	Sinks, Taps And Fixtures Cleaned And Disinfected										
27	Clean And Disinfect Cabinets And Units										
28	Feminine Hygiene Dispensers Re-Stocked										
29	Feminine Hygiene Bins/Containers Emptied And Cleared										

Care Home Cleaning Tasks - Toilet & Restroom	M	T	W	T	F	S	S	Cleaned By	Checked By	Date/Time
Clean & Vacuum Central Heating Units (Backs Of Radiators)										
Wash And Clean Ceiling Light Covers										
Toilet Roll Holders And Toilet Rolls Re-Stocked										
Toilet Roll Holders Cleaned And Disinfected										
Clean Inside The Toilets And Urinals With Disinfectant										
Toilet Seats Cleaned And Disinfected										
Clean Top Of Toilets Tanks, The Bases And Behind Toilets										
Urinal Handles Cleaned And Disinfected										
Urinal Screens Cleaned, Disinfected And Blocks Replaced										
Paper Dispensers And Paper Towel Rolls Re-Stocked										
Paper Dispensers And Paper Towel Roll Cleaned & Disinfected										
The Floors Are Swept And Free From Debris And Litter										
Floors Mopped Clean With Cleaning Or Disinfecting Solution										
Put Up Or Place Wet Floor Signs After Mopping Floors										
Showers And Shower Heads, Cleaned And Disinfected										
Soak Shower Heads										
Clean And Disinfect Glass Shower Doors/Outer Doors										
Clean Soap Scum From Shower Walls										
Clean Blinds (Dust The Blinds With A Damp Microfibre Cloth)										
Clean Curtains (Vacuum On A Low Setting Or Wash If Possible)										
Dust And Wash Radiator Covers										
Clean And Disinfect Commodes Between Each Use										
Clean And Disinfect Shower Chairs Between Each Use										
Bath Hoists Cleaned And Disinfected Between Each Use										
Scrub Tub/Bath, Polish Facets And Taps, Clean & Disinfected										
Toothbrush Holders And Soap Holders Cleaned										
Re-Place Shower Curtains With Clean Fresh Ones										
Wash And Clean Air Vents										
Thoroughly Clean Grout And Tiles										
Disinfect And Clean All The Walls From Top To Bottom										
Wash And Clean Windows (Inside And Outside)										
Unclog The Drains (Sink, Bath And Shower)										
Pour Drain Cleaner Down Sink, Shower & Bath Drains										
Floor Drains And Drain Covers Are Open And Free Of Debris										
Hair Dryers Cleaned And Disinfected And Operating Correctly										
Light Bulbs Checked And None Functioning Bulbs Replaced										
Check Hardware, Door Stops And Lock Mechanisms										

CARE HOME BEDROOM CLEANING *Checklist*

Building	Location	Room Number	Area

Start Date & Time	Finnish Date & Time	Name	Signature

	Care Home Cleaning Tasks - Bedrooms	M	T	W	T	F	S	S	Cleaned By	Checked By	Date/Time
1	Clean And Sanitize All The Desks And Tables										
2	Clean And Sanitize All The Counter Tops And Surface Areas										
3	Wipe Down The Walls Wherever There Are Spills And Splashes										
4	Disinfect Touch Points, Light Switches And Other Switches										
5	Clean And Disinfect All Doors, Handles And Doorknobs										
6	Clean And Dust Door Frames, Remember To Dust The Tops										
7	Dust Light Fixtures With A Duster Or A Microfibre Cloth										
8	Clean & Wipe Mirrors Remove Fingerprints, Smears & Dirt										
9	Clean And Dust Bedside Cabinets										
10	Clean And Sanitize Over Chair Tables										
11	Clean And Sanitize Over Bed Tables										
12	Clean And Check Bed Frames										
13	Mattresses Hoovered And Cleaned With Disinfectant										
14	Clean And Polish Bookshelves, Remember To Dust The Top										
15	Remove, Wash And Clean Any Dirty Cups Or Glasses										
16	Remove, Wash And Clean Any Dirty Plates, Bowels Or Cutlery										
17	Clean And Sanitize Any Chairs And Seats										
18	Water Jug (Washed Thoroughly Each Day & Re-Filled)										
19	Water Any Plants And Flowers										
20	Dust Plant Leafs (A Healthy Plant Needs To Be Clear Of Dust)										
21	Empty The Waste Basket And Recycling Bin										
22	Clean And Disinfectant The Waste Bin And Recycling Bin										
23	Clean And Wipe Down Windowsills										
24	Spray Air Freshener This Keeps The Room Smelling Fresh										
25	Clean And Disinfect Cabinets And Units										
26	Clean And Sanitize Desk Accessories										
27	Replace Dirty Linen And Move To Laundry Room										
28	Polish Any Wooden Furniture And Hardwood Surfaces										
29	Clean Skirting Boards/Baseboards And Corners										

Care Home Cleaning Tasks - Bedrooms Continued	M	T	W	T	F	S	S	Cleaned By	Checked By	Date/Time
Dust Television, Top Sides And Back, TV Unit And TV Stand										
Clean TV Screen With Soft Damp Cloth (Use Water/Cleaner)										
Vacuum/Hoover Between Bedroom Furniture And The Walls										
Clean And Sanitize Resident's Personal Wheelchair										
Check For Broken Wheelchairs, Frames and Wheels										
Vacuum Under Furniture, Beds, Sofas and Dressers										
Vacuum And Hoover The Carpets, Mats And Rugs										
Vacuum Furnishings, Cushions, Chairs, Sofas And Couches										
Steam Clean Carpets And Rugs										
Dust And Clean Any Picture Frames And Photo Frames										
Ledges, Flat Surfaces And The Tops Of Wardrobes Dusted										
Clean & Check Contents Of Medicine Trolleys & Cupboards										
Clean And Sanitize Mobile Phone, Phone Case And Screen										
Clean & Vacuum The Desk Chair, Legs And Chair Wheels										
Wash And Clean Air Vents										
Dust Ceiling Fan Blades With Duster Or A Microfibre Cloth										
Wash And Clean Windows (Inside And Outside)										
Dust And Clean The Walls From Top To Bottom										
Clean Blinds (Dust The Blinds With A Damp Microfibre Cloth)										
Clean Curtains (Vacuum On A Low Setting Or Wash If Possible)										
Dust And Wash Radiator Covers										
Wash And Clean Ceiling Light Covers										
Clean & Vacuum Central Heating Units (Backs Of Radiators)										
Clean And Disinfect Any Handrails										
Hand Towels Replaced With Fresh Clean Ones										
Sink Wall Mirror Cleaned With Glass Cleaner										
Sinks, Taps And Fixtures Cleaned And Disinfected										
Pour Drain Cleaner Down Sink Drains										
Check For Broken Furniture (Report/Schedule Maintenance)										
Light Bulbs Checked And None Functioning Bulbs Replaced										
Check Hardware, Door Stops And Lock Mechanisms										
Fire Exit Lights And Emergency Lights Checked & Functioning										
Test Carbon Monoxide Alarm And Replace Batteries If Required										
Test Smoke Detector Alarm And Replace Batteries If Required										
Paper Dispensers And Paper Towel Rolls Re-Stocked										
Soap Dispensers, Hand Sanitizers And Hand Gels Are Refilled										
Face Masks, Protective Gloves And Face Shields Re-Stocked										

CARE HOME COMMUNAL AREA CLEANING *Checklist*

Building	Location	Room Number	Area

Start Date & Time	Finnish Date & Time	Name	Signature

	Care Home Cleaning Tasks - Communal Area	M	T	W	T	F	S	S	Cleaned By	Checked By	Date/Time
1	Clean And Sanitize All The Desks And Tables										
2	Clean And Sanitize All The Counter Tops And Surface Areas										
3	Wipe Down The Walls Wherever There Are Spills And Splashes										
4	Disinfect Touch Points, Light Switches And Other Switches										
5	Clean And Disinfect All Doors, Handles And Doorknobs										
6	Clean And Dust Door Frames, Remember To Dust The Tops										
7	Dust Light Fixtures & Shades With A Duster Or A Microfibre Cloth										
8	Clean And Wipe Mirrors Remove Fingerprints, Smears & Dirt										
9	Clean And Sanitize Over Chair Tables										
10	Clean And Polish Bookshelves, Remember To Dust The Top										
11	Remove, Wash And Clean Any Dirty Cups Or Glasses										
12	Remove, Wash And Clean Any Dirty Plates, Bowels Or Cutlery										
13	Clean And Sanitize Any Chairs, Seats And Benches										
14	Water Jugs (Washed Thoroughly Each Day & Re-Filled)										
15	Water Any Plants And Flowers										
16	Dust Plant Leafs (A Healthy Plant Needs To Be Clear Of Dust)										
17	Empty The Waste Baskets And Recycling Bins										
18	Clean And Disinfectant The Waste Bins And Recycling Bins										
19	Clean And Wipe Down Windowsills										
20	Spray Air Freshener This Keeps The Room Smelling Fresh										
21	Clean And Disinfect Cabinets And Units										
22	Clean And Sanitize Desk Accessories										
23	Replace Dirty Table Linen And Move To Laundry Room										
24	Polish Any Wooden Furniture And Hardwood Surfaces										
25	Clean Skirting Boards/Baseboards And Corners										
26	Clean And Polish Fireplace Mantelpiece And Surrounds										
27	Wipe Down Equipment & Sanitize Tea And Coffee Making Facilities										
28	Clean And Sanitize Telephones, Cords/Leads & All Touch Points										
29	Clean And Sanitize Walking Sticks And Any Other Walking Aids										

Care Home Cleaning Tasks - Communal Area	M	T	W	T	F	S	S	Cleaned By	Checked By	Date/Time
Dust Television, Top Sides And Back, TV Unit And TV Stand										
Clean TV Screen With Soft Damp Cloth (Use Water/Cleaner)										
Vacuum/Hoover Between Furniture And The Walls										
Clean And Sanitize All Wheelchairs										
Check For Broken Wheelchairs, Frames and Wheels										
Vacuum Under Furniture, Units, Tables And Cabinets										
Vacuum And Hoover The Carpets, Mats And Rugs										
Vacuum Furnishings, Cushions, Chairs, Sofas And Couches										
Steam Clean Carpets And Rugs										
Dust And Clean Any Picture Frames And Wall Art										
Clean & Check Contents Of Medicine Trolleys & Cupboards										
Clean & Vacuum The Desk Chair, Legs And Chair Wheels										
Wash And Clean Air Vents										
Dust Ceiling Fan Blades With Duster Or A Microfibre Cloth										
Wash And Clean Windows (Inside And Outside)										
Dust And Clean The Walls From Top To Bottom										
Clean Blinds (Dust The Blinds With A Damp Microfibre Cloth)										
Clean Curtains (Vacuum On A Low Setting Or Wash If Possible)										
Dust And Wash Radiator Covers										
Wash And Clean Ceiling Light Covers										
Clean & Vacuum Central Heating Units (Backs Of Radiators)										
Clean And Disinfect Any Handrails										
Clean And Sanitize Computer, Keyboard And Computer Mice										
Clean And Sanitize iPads, Tablets, Laptops & Mobile Phones										
Floors Mopped Clean With Cleaning Or Disinfecting Solution										
The Floors Are Swept And Free From Debris And Litter										
Clean Sliding Doors and Room Partitions										
Throw Away Outdated Newspapers, Magazines, Papers										
Check For Broken Furniture (Report/Schedule Maintenance)										
Light Bulbs Checked And None Functioning Bulbs Replaced										
Check Hardware, Door Stops And Lock Mechanisms										
Fire Exit Lights And Emergency Lights Checked & Functioning										
Test Carbon Monoxide Alarm And Replace Batteries If Required										
Test Smoke Detector Alarm And Replace Batteries If Required										
Paper Dispensers And Paper Towel Rolls Re-Stocked										
Soap Dispensers, Hand Sanitizers And Hand Gels Are Refilled										
Face Masks, Protective Gloves And Face Shields Re-Stocked										

CARE HOME TOILET & RESTROOM CLEANING *Checklis*

Building	Location	Room Number	Area

Start Date & Time	Finnish Date & Time	Name	Signature

	Care Home Cleaning Tasks - Toilet & Restroom	M	T	W	T	F	S	S	Cleaned By	Checked By	Date/Tim
1	Clean And Sanitize All The Counter Tops And Surface Areas										
2	Wipe Down The Walls Wherever There Are Spills And Splashes										
3	Disinfect Touch Points, Light Switches And Other Switches										
4	Clean And Disinfect All Doors, Handles And Doorknobs										
5	Clean And Dust Door Frames, Remember To Dust The Tops										
6	Dust Light Fixtures With A Duster Or A Microfibre Cloth										
7	Wall Mirrors Cleaned With Glass Cleaner										
8	Clean Any Bathroom Glasses And Cups										
9	Clean And Sanitize Any Chairs And Seats										
10	Empty The Waste Basket And Recycling Bin										
11	Clean And Disinfectant The Waste Bin And Recycling Bin										
12	Clean And Wipe Down Windowsills										
13	Spray Air Freshener This Keeps The Room Smelling Fresh										
14	Air/Odour Control Systems Are Filled And Operating Correctly										
15	Clean Skirting Boards/Baseboards And Corners										
16	Vacuum And Hoover Bath Mats, Shower Mats And Rugs										
17	Replace Bath Mats, Shower Mats And Rugs With Clean Ones										
18	Steam Clean Carpets And Rugs										
19	Hand Towels Replaced With Fresh Clean Ones										
20	Bath Towels Replaced With Fresh Clean Ones										
21	Face Towels Replaced With Fresh Clean Ones										
22	Electric Hand Dryers Cleaned, Disinfected & Operating Correctly										
23	Soap Dispensers, Sanitizers And Hand Gels Are Refilled										
24	Clean & Check Contents Of Medicine Trolleys & Cupboards										
25	Clean And Disinfect Any Handrails										
26	Sinks, Taps And Fixtures Cleaned And Disinfected										
27	Clean And Disinfect Cabinets And Units										
28	Feminine Hygiene Dispensers Re-Stocked										
29	Feminine Hygiene Bins/Containers Emptied And Cleared										

Care Home Cleaning Tasks - Toilet & Restroom	M	T	W	T	F	S	S	Cleaned By	Checked By	Date/Time
30 Clean & Vacuum Central Heating Units (Backs Of Radiators)										
31 Wash And Clean Ceiling Light Covers										
32 Toilet Roll Holders And Toilet Rolls Re-Stocked										
33 Toilet Roll Holders Cleaned And Disinfected										
34 Clean Inside The Toilets And Urinals With Disinfectant										
35 Toilet Seats Cleaned And Disinfected										
36 Clean Top Of Toilets Tanks, The Bases And Behind Toilets										
37 Urinal Handles Cleaned And Disinfected										
38 Urinal Screens Cleaned, Disinfected And Blocks Replaced										
39 Paper Dispensers And Paper Towel Rolls Re-Stocked										
40 Paper Dispensers And Paper Towel Roll Cleaned & Disinfected										
41 The Floors Are Swept And Free From Debris And Litter										
42 Floors Mopped Clean With Cleaning Or Disinfecting Solution										
43 Put Up Or Place Wet Floor Signs After Mopping Floors										
44 Showers And Shower Heads, Cleaned And Disinfected										
45 Soak Shower Heads										
46 Clean And Disinfect Glass Shower Doors/Outer Doors										
47 Clean Soap Scum From Shower Walls										
48 Clean Blinds (Dust The Blinds With A Damp Microfibre Cloth)										
49 Clean Curtains (Vacuum On A Low Setting Or Wash If Possible)										
50 Dust And Wash Radiator Covers										
51 Clean And Disinfect Commodes Between Each Use										
52 Clean And Disinfect Shower Chairs Between Each Use										
53 Bath Hoists Cleaned And Disinfected Between Each Use										
54 Scrub Tub/Bath, Polish Facets And Taps, Clean & Disinfected										
55 Toothbrush Holders And Soap Holders Cleaned										
56 Re-Place Shower Curtains With Clean Fresh Ones										
57 Wash And Clean Air Vents										
Thoroughly Clean Grout And Tiles										
Disinfect And Clean All The Walls From Top To Bottom										
Wash And Clean Windows (Inside And Outside)										
Unclog The Drains (Sink, Bath And Shower)										
Pour Drain Cleaner Down Sink, Shower & Bath Drains										
Floor Drains And Drain Covers Are Open And Free Of Debris										
Hair Dryers Cleaned And Disinfected And Operating Correctly										
Light Bulbs Checked And None Functioning Bulbs Replaced										
Check Hardware, Door Stops And Lock Mechanisms										

CARE HOME BEDROOM CLEANING *Checklist*

Building	Location	Room Number	Area

Start Date & Time	Finnish Date & Time	Name	Signature

	Care Home Cleaning Tasks - Bedrooms	M	T	W	T	F	S	S	Cleaned By	Checked By	Date/Tim
1	Clean And Sanitize All The Desks And Tables										
2	Clean And Sanitize All The Counter Tops And Surface Areas										
3	Wipe Down The Walls Wherever There Are Spills And Splashes										
4	Disinfect Touch Points, Light Switches And Other Switches										
5	Clean And Disinfect All Doors, Handles And Doorknobs										
6	Clean And Dust Door Frames, Remember To Dust The Tops										
7	Dust Light Fixtures With A Duster Or A Microfibre Cloth										
8	Clean & Wipe Mirrors Remove Fingerprints, Smears & Dirt										
9	Clean And Dust Bedside Cabinets										
10	Clean And Sanitize Over Chair Tables										
11	Clean And Sanitize Over Bed Tables										
12	Clean And Check Bed Frames										
13	Mattresses Hoovered And Cleaned With Disinfectant										
14	Clean And Polish Bookshelves, Remember To Dust The Top										
15	Remove, Wash And Clean Any Dirty Cups Or Glasses										
16	Remove, Wash And Clean Any Dirty Plates, Bowels Or Cutlery										
17	Clean And Sanitize Any Chairs And Seats										
18	Water Jug (Washed Thoroughly Each Day & Re-Filled)										
19	Water Any Plants And Flowers										
20	Dust Plant Leafs (A Healthy Plant Needs To Be Clear Of Dust)										
21	Empty The Waste Basket And Recycling Bin										
22	Clean And Disinfectant The Waste Bin And Recycling Bin										
23	Clean And Wipe Down Windowsills										
24	Spray Air Freshener This Keeps The Room Smelling Fresh										
25	Clean And Disinfect Cabinets And Units										
26	Clean And Sanitize Desk Accessories										
27	Replace Dirty Linen And Move To Laundry Room										
28	Polish Any Wooden Furniture And Hardwood Surfaces										
29	Clean Skirting Boards/Baseboards And Corners										

Care Home Cleaning Tasks - Bedrooms Continued	M	T	W	T	F	S	S	Cleaned By	Checked By	Date/Time
Dust Television, Top Sides And Back, TV Unit And TV Stand										
Clean TV Screen With Soft Damp Cloth (Use Water/Cleaner)										
Vacuum/Hoover Between Bedroom Furniture And The Walls										
Clean And Sanitize Resident's Personal Wheelchair										
Check For Broken Wheelchairs, Frames and Wheels										
Vacuum Under Furniture, Beds, Sofas and Dressers										
Vacuum And Hoover The Carpets, Mats And Rugs										
Vacuum Furnishings, Cushions, Chairs, Sofas And Couches										
Steam Clean Carpets And Rugs										
Dust And Clean Any Picture Frames And Photo Frames										
Ledges, Flat Surfaces And The Tops Of Wardrobes Dusted										
Clean & Check Contents Of Medicine Trolleys & Cupboards										
Clean And Sanitize Mobile Phone, Phone Case And Screen										
Clean & Vacuum The Desk Chair, Legs And Chair Wheels										
Wash And Clean Air Vents										
Dust Ceiling Fan Blades With Duster Or A Microfibre Cloth										
Wash And Clean Windows (Inside And Outside)										
Dust And Clean The Walls From Top To Bottom										
Clean Blinds (Dust The Blinds With A Damp Microfibre Cloth)										
Clean Curtains (Vacuum On A Low Setting Or Wash If Possible)										
Dust And Wash Radiator Covers										
Wash And Clean Ceiling Light Covers										
Clean & Vacuum Central Heating Units (Backs Of Radiators)										
Clean And Disinfect Any Handrails										
Hand Towels Replaced With Fresh Clean Ones										
Sink Wall Mirror Cleaned With Glass Cleaner										
Sinks, Taps And Fixtures Cleaned And Disinfected										
Pour Drain Cleaner Down Sink Drains										
Check For Broken Furniture (Report/Schedule Maintenance)										
Light Bulbs Checked And None Functioning Bulbs Replaced										
Check Hardware, Door Stops And Lock Mechanisms										
Fire Exit Lights And Emergency Lights Checked & Functioning										
Test Carbon Monoxide Alarm And Replace Batteries If Required										
Test Smoke Detector Alarm And Replace Batteries If Required										
Paper Dispensers And Paper Towel Rolls Re-Stocked										
Soap Dispensers, Hand Sanitizers And Hand Gels Are Refilled										
Face Masks, Protective Gloves And Face Shields Re-Stocked										

CARE HOME COMMUNAL AREA CLEANING *Checklist*

Building	Location	Room Number	Area

Start Date & Time	Finnish Date & Time	Name	Signature

	Care Home Cleaning Tasks - Communal Area	M	T	W	T	F	S	S	Cleaned By	Checked By	Date/Tim
1	Clean And Sanitize All The Desks And Tables										
2	Clean And Sanitize All The Counter Tops And Surface Areas										
3	Wipe Down The Walls Wherever There Are Spills And Splashes										
4	Disinfect Touch Points, Light Switches And Other Switches										
5	Clean And Disinfect All Doors, Handles And Doorknobs										
6	Clean And Dust Door Frames, Remember To Dust The Tops										
7	Dust Light Fixtures & Shades With A Duster Or A Microfibre Cloth										
8	Clean And Wipe Mirrors Remove Fingerprints, Smears & Dirt										
9	Clean And Sanitize Over Chair Tables										
10	Clean And Polish Bookshelves, Remember To Dust The Top										
11	Remove, Wash And Clean Any Dirty Cups Or Glasses										
12	Remove, Wash And Clean Any Dirty Plates, Bowels Or Cutlery										
13	Clean And Sanitize Any Chairs, Seats And Benches										
14	Water Jugs (Washed Thoroughly Each Day & Re-Filled)										
15	Water Any Plants And Flowers										
16	Dust Plant Leafs (A Healthy Plant Needs To Be Clear Of Dust)										
17	Empty The Waste Baskets And Recycling Bins										
18	Clean And Disinfectant The Waste Bins And Recycling Bins										
19	Clean And Wipe Down Windowsills										
20	Spray Air Freshener This Keeps The Room Smelling Fresh										
21	Clean And Disinfect Cabinets And Units										
22	Clean And Sanitize Desk Accessories										
23	Replace Dirty Table Linen And Move To Laundry Room										
24	Polish Any Wooden Furniture And Hardwood Surfaces										
25	Clean Skirting Boards/Baseboards And Corners										
26	Clean And Polish Fireplace Mantelpiece And Surrounds										
27	Wipe Down Equipment & Sanitize Tea And Coffee Making Facilities										
28	Clean And Sanitize Telephones, Cords/Leads & All Touch Points										
29	Clean And Sanitize Walking Sticks And Any Other Walking Aids										

Care Home Cleaning Tasks - Communal Area	M	T	W	T	F	S	S	Cleaned By	Checked By	Date/Time
Dust Television, Top Sides And Back, TV Unit And TV Stand										
Clean TV Screen With Soft Damp Cloth (Use Water/Cleaner)										
Vacuum/Hoover Between Furniture And The Walls										
Clean And Sanitize All Wheelchairs										
Check For Broken Wheelchairs, Frames and Wheels										
Vacuum Under Furniture, Units, Tables And Cabinets										
Vacuum And Hoover The Carpets, Mats And Rugs										
Vacuum Furnishings, Cushions, Chairs, Sofas And Couches										
Steam Clean Carpets And Rugs										
Dust And Clean Any Picture Frames And Wall Art										
Clean & Check Contents Of Medicine Trolleys & Cupboards										
Clean & Vacuum The Desk Chair, Legs And Chair Wheels										
Wash And Clean Air Vents										
Dust Ceiling Fan Blades With Duster Or A Microfibre Cloth										
Wash And Clean Windows (Inside And Outside)										
Dust And Clean The Walls From Top To Bottom										
Clean Blinds (Dust The Blinds With A Damp Microfibre Cloth)										
Clean Curtains (Vacuum On A Low Setting Or Wash If Possible)										
Dust And Wash Radiator Covers										
Wash And Clean Ceiling Light Covers										
Clean & Vacuum Central Heating Units (Backs Of Radiators)										
Clean And Disinfect Any Handrails										
Clean And Sanitize Computer, Keyboard And Computer Mice										
Clean And Sanitize iPads, Tablets, Laptops & Mobile Phones										
Floors Mopped Clean With Cleaning Or Disinfecting Solution										
The Floors Are Swept And Free From Debris And Litter										
Clean Sliding Doors and Room Partitions										
Throw Away Outdated Newspapers, Magazines, Papers										
Check For Broken Furniture (Report/Schedule Maintenance)										
Light Bulbs Checked And None Functioning Bulbs Replaced										
Check Hardware, Door Stops And Lock Mechanisms										
Fire Exit Lights And Emergency Lights Checked & Functioning										
Test Carbon Monoxide Alarm And Replace Batteries If Required										
Test Smoke Detector Alarm And Replace Batteries If Required										
Paper Dispensers And Paper Towel Rolls Re-Stocked										
Soap Dispensers, Hand Sanitizers And Hand Gels Are Refilled										
Face Masks, Protective Gloves And Face Shields Re-Stocked										

CARE HOME TOILET & RESTROOM CLEANING *Checklist*

Building	Location	Room Number	Area

Start Date & Time	Finnish Date & Time	Name	Signature

	Care Home Cleaning Tasks - Toilet & Restroom	M	T	W	T	F	S	S	Cleaned By	Checked By	Date/Time
1	Clean And Sanitize All The Counter Tops And Surface Areas										
2	Wipe Down The Walls Wherever There Are Spills And Splashes										
3	Disinfect Touch Points, Light Switches And Other Switches										
4	Clean And Disinfect All Doors, Handles And Doorknobs										
5	Clean And Dust Door Frames, Remember To Dust The Tops										
6	Dust Light Fixtures With A Duster Or A Microfibre Cloth										
7	Wall Mirrors Cleaned With Glass Cleaner										
8	Clean Any Bathroom Glasses And Cups										
9	Clean And Sanitize Any Chairs And Seats										
10	Empty The Waste Basket And Recycling Bin										
11	Clean And Disinfectant The Waste Bin And Recycling Bin										
12	Clean And Wipe Down Windowsills										
13	Spray Air Freshener This Keeps The Room Smelling Fresh										
14	Air/Odour Control Systems Are Filled And Operating Correctly										
15	Clean Skirting Boards/Baseboards And Corners										
16	Vacuum And Hoover Bath Mats, Shower Mats And Rugs										
17	Replace Bath Mats, Shower Mats And Rugs With Clean Ones										
18	Steam Clean Carpets And Rugs										
19	Hand Towels Replaced With Fresh Clean Ones										
20	Bath Towels Replaced With Fresh Clean Ones										
21	Face Towels Replaced With Fresh Clean Ones										
22	Electric Hand Dryers Cleaned, Disinfected & Operating Correctly										
23	Soap Dispensers, Sanitizers And Hand Gels Are Refilled										
24	Clean & Check Contents Of Medicine Trolleys & Cupboards										
25	Clean And Disinfect Any Handrails										
26	Sinks, Taps And Fixtures Cleaned And Disinfected										
27	Clean And Disinfect Cabinets And Units										
28	Feminine Hygiene Dispensers Re-Stocked										
29	Feminine Hygiene Bins/Containers Emptied And Cleared										

Care Home Cleaning Tasks - Toilet & Restroom	M	T	W	T	F	S	S	Cleaned By	Checked By	Date/Time
Clean & Vacuum Central Heating Units (Backs Of Radiators)										
Wash And Clean Ceiling Light Covers										
Toilet Roll Holders And Toilet Rolls Re-Stocked										
Toilet Roll Holders Cleaned And Disinfected										
Clean Inside The Toilets And Urinals With Disinfectant										
Toilet Seats Cleaned And Disinfected										
Clean Top Of Toilets Tanks, The Bases And Behind Toilets										
Urinal Handles Cleaned And Disinfected										
Urinal Screens Cleaned, Disinfected And Blocks Replaced										
Paper Dispensers And Paper Towel Rolls Re-Stocked										
Paper Dispensers And Paper Towel Roll Cleaned & Disinfected										
The Floors Are Swept And Free From Debris And Litter										
Floors Mopped Clean With Cleaning Or Disinfecting Solution										
Put Up Or Place Wet Floor Signs After Mopping Floors										
Showers And Shower Heads, Cleaned And Disinfected										
Soak Shower Heads										
Clean And Disinfect Glass Shower Doors/Outer Doors										
Clean Soap Scum From Shower Walls										
Clean Blinds (Dust The Blinds With A Damp Microfibre Cloth)										
Clean Curtains (Vacuum On A Low Setting Or Wash If Possible)										
Dust And Wash Radiator Covers										
Clean And Disinfect Commodes Between Each Use										
Clean And Disinfect Shower Chairs Between Each Use										
Bath Hoists Cleaned And Disinfected Between Each Use										
Scrub Tub/Bath, Polish Facets And Taps, Clean & Disinfected										
Toothbrush Holders And Soap Holders Cleaned										
Re-Place Shower Curtains With Clean Fresh Ones										
Wash And Clean Air Vents										
Thoroughly Clean Grout And Tiles										
Disinfect And Clean All The Walls From Top To Bottom										
Wash And Clean Windows (Inside And Outside)										
Unclog The Drains (Sink, Bath And Shower)										
Pour Drain Cleaner Down Sink, Shower & Bath Drains										
Floor Drains And Drain Covers Are Open And Free Of Debris										
Hair Dryers Cleaned And Disinfected And Operating Correctly										
Light Bulbs Checked And None Functioning Bulbs Replaced										
Check Hardware, Door Stops And Lock Mechanisms										

CARE HOME BEDROOM CLEANING *Checklist*

Building	Location	Room Number	Area

Start Date & Time	Finnish Date & Time	Name	Signature

	Care Home Cleaning Tasks - Bedrooms	M	T	W	T	F	S	S	Cleaned By	Checked By	Date/Tim
1	Clean And Sanitize All The Desks And Tables										
2	Clean And Sanitize All The Counter Tops And Surface Areas										
3	Wipe Down The Walls Wherever There Are Spills And Splashes										
4	Disinfect Touch Points, Light Switches And Other Switches										
5	Clean And Disinfect All Doors, Handles And Doorknobs										
6	Clean And Dust Door Frames, Remember To Dust The Tops										
7	Dust Light Fixtures With A Duster Or A Microfibre Cloth										
8	Clean & Wipe Mirrors Remove Fingerprints, Smears & Dirt										
9	Clean And Dust Bedside Cabinets										
10	Clean And Sanitize Over Chair Tables										
11	Clean And Sanitize Over Bed Tables										
12	Clean And Check Bed Frames										
13	Mattresses Hoovered And Cleaned With Disinfectant										
14	Clean And Polish Bookshelves, Remember To Dust The Top										
15	Remove, Wash And Clean Any Dirty Cups Or Glasses										
16	Remove, Wash And Clean Any Dirty Plates, Bowels Or Cutlery										
17	Clean And Sanitize Any Chairs And Seats										
18	Water Jug (Washed Thoroughly Each Day & Re-Filled)										
19	Water Any Plants And Flowers										
20	Dust Plant Leafs (A Healthy Plant Needs To Be Clear Of Dust)										
21	Empty The Waste Basket And Recycling Bin										
22	Clean And Disinfectant The Waste Bin And Recycling Bin										
23	Clean And Wipe Down Windowsills										
24	Spray Air Freshener This Keeps The Room Smelling Fresh										
25	Clean And Disinfect Cabinets And Units										
26	Clean And Sanitize Desk Accessories										
27	Replace Dirty Linen And Move To Laundry Room										
28	Polish Any Wooden Furniture And Hardwood Surfaces										
29	Clean Skirting Boards/Baseboards And Corners										

Care Home Cleaning Tasks - Bedrooms Continued	M	T	W	T	F	S	S	Cleaned By	Checked By	Date/Time
Dust Television, Top Sides And Back, TV Unit And TV Stand										
Clean TV Screen With Soft Damp Cloth (Use Water/Cleaner)										
Vacuum/Hoover Between Bedroom Furniture And The Walls										
Clean And Sanitize Resident's Personal Wheelchair										
Check For Broken Wheelchairs, Frames and Wheels										
Vacuum Under Furniture, Beds, Sofas and Dressers										
Vacuum And Hoover The Carpets, Mats And Rugs										
Vacuum Furnishings, Cushions, Chairs, Sofas And Couches										
Steam Clean Carpets And Rugs										
Dust And Clean Any Picture Frames And Photo Frames										
Ledges, Flat Surfaces And The Tops Of Wardrobes Dusted										
Clean & Check Contents Of Medicine Trolleys & Cupboards										
Clean And Sanitize Mobile Phone, Phone Case And Screen										
Clean & Vacuum The Desk Chair, Legs And Chair Wheels										
Wash And Clean Air Vents										
Dust Ceiling Fan Blades With Duster Or A Microfibre Cloth										
Wash And Clean Windows (Inside And Outside)										
Dust And Clean The Walls From Top To Bottom										
Clean Blinds (Dust The Blinds With A Damp Microfibre Cloth)										
Clean Curtains (Vacuum On A Low Setting Or Wash If Possible)										
Dust And Wash Radiator Covers										
Wash And Clean Ceiling Light Covers										
Clean & Vacuum Central Heating Units (Backs Of Radiators)										
Clean And Disinfect Any Handrails										
Hand Towels Replaced With Fresh Clean Ones										
Sink Wall Mirror Cleaned With Glass Cleaner										
Sinks, Taps And Fixtures Cleaned And Disinfected										
Pour Drain Cleaner Down Sink Drains										
Check For Broken Furniture (Report/Schedule Maintenance)										
Light Bulbs Checked And None Functioning Bulbs Replaced										
Check Hardware, Door Stops And Lock Mechanisms										
Fire Exit Lights And Emergency Lights Checked & Functioning										
Test Carbon Monoxide Alarm And Replace Batteries If Required										
Test Smoke Detector Alarm And Replace Batteries If Required										
Paper Dispensers And Paper Towel Rolls Re-Stocked										
Soap Dispensers, Hand Sanitizers And Hand Gels Are Refilled										
Face Masks, Protective Gloves And Face Shields Re-Stocked										

CARE HOME COMMUNAL AREA CLEANING *Checklist*

Building	Location	Room Number	Area

Start Date & Time	Finnish Date & Time	Name	Signature

	Care Home Cleaning Tasks - Communal Area	M	T	W	T	F	S	S	Cleaned By	Checked By	Date/Tim
1	Clean And Sanitize All The Desks And Tables										
2	Clean And Sanitize All The Counter Tops And Surface Areas										
3	Wipe Down The Walls Wherever There Are Spills And Splashes										
4	Disinfect Touch Points, Light Switches And Other Switches										
5	Clean And Disinfect All Doors, Handles And Doorknobs										
6	Clean And Dust Door Frames, Remember To Dust The Tops										
7	Dust Light Fixtures & Shades With A Duster Or A Microfibre Cloth										
8	Clean And Wipe Mirrors Remove Fingerprints, Smears & Dirt										
9	Clean And Sanitize Over Chair Tables										
10	Clean And Polish Bookshelves, Remember To Dust The Top										
11	Remove, Wash And Clean Any Dirty Cups Or Glasses										
12	Remove, Wash And Clean Any Dirty Plates, Bowels Or Cutlery										
13	Clean And Sanitize Any Chairs, Seats And Benches										
14	Water Jugs (Washed Thoroughly Each Day & Re-Filled)										
15	Water Any Plants And Flowers										
16	Dust Plant Leafs (A Healthy Plant Needs To Be Clear Of Dust)										
17	Empty The Waste Baskets And Recycling Bins										
18	Clean And Disinfectant The Waste Bins And Recycling Bins										
19	Clean And Wipe Down Windowsills										
20	Spray Air Freshener This Keeps The Room Smelling Fresh										
21	Clean And Disinfect Cabinets And Units										
22	Clean And Sanitize Desk Accessories										
23	Replace Dirty Table Linen And Move To Laundry Room										
24	Polish Any Wooden Furniture And Hardwood Surfaces										
25	Clean Skirting Boards/Baseboards And Corners										
26	Clean And Polish Fireplace Mantelpiece And Surrounds										
27	Wipe Down Equipment & Sanitize Tea And Coffee Making Facilities										
28	Clean And Sanitize Telephones, Cords/Leads & All Touch Points										
29	Clean And Sanitize Walking Sticks And Any Other Walking Aids										

Care Home Cleaning Tasks - Communal Area	M	T	W	T	F	S	S	Cleaned By	Checked By	Date/Time
Dust Television, Top Sides And Back, TV Unit And TV Stand										
Clean TV Screen With Soft Damp Cloth (Use Water/Cleaner)										
Vacuum/Hoover Between Furniture And The Walls										
Clean And Sanitize All Wheelchairs										
Check For Broken Wheelchairs, Frames and Wheels										
Vacuum Under Furniture, Units, Tables And Cabinets										
Vacuum And Hoover The Carpets, Mats And Rugs										
Vacuum Furnishings, Cushions, Chairs, Sofas And Couches										
Steam Clean Carpets And Rugs										
Dust And Clean Any Picture Frames And Wall Art										
Clean & Check Contents Of Medicine Trolleys & Cupboards										
Clean & Vacuum The Desk Chair, Legs And Chair Wheels										
Wash And Clean Air Vents										
Dust Ceiling Fan Blades With Duster Or A Microfibre Cloth										
Wash And Clean Windows (Inside And Outside)										
Dust And Clean The Walls From Top To Bottom										
Clean Blinds (Dust The Blinds With A Damp Microfibre Cloth)										
Clean Curtains (Vacuum On A Low Setting Or Wash If Possible)										
Dust And Wash Radiator Covers										
Wash And Clean Ceiling Light Covers										
Clean & Vacuum Central Heating Units (Backs Of Radiators)										
Clean And Disinfect Any Handrails										
Clean And Sanitize Computer, Keyboard And Computer Mice										
Clean And Sanitize iPads, Tablets, Laptops & Mobile Phones										
Floors Mopped Clean With Cleaning Or Disinfecting Solution										
The Floors Are Swept And Free From Debris And Litter										
Clean Sliding Doors and Room Partitions										
Throw Away Outdated Newspapers, Magazines, Papers										
Check For Broken Furniture (Report/Schedule Maintenance)										
Light Bulbs Checked And None Functioning Bulbs Replaced										
Check Hardware, Door Stops And Lock Mechanisms										
Fire Exit Lights And Emergency Lights Checked & Functioning										
Test Carbon Monoxide Alarm And Replace Batteries If Required										
Test Smoke Detector Alarm And Replace Batteries If Required										
Paper Dispensers And Paper Towel Rolls Re-Stocked										
Soap Dispensers, Hand Sanitizers And Hand Gels Are Refilled										
Face Masks, Protective Gloves And Face Shields Re-Stocked										

CARE HOME TOILET & RESTROOM CLEANING *Checklist*

Building	Location	Room Number	Area

Start Date & Time	Finnish Date & Time	Name	Signature

	Care Home Cleaning Tasks - Toilet & Restroom	M	T	W	T	F	S	S	Cleaned By	Checked By	Date/Time
1	Clean And Sanitize All The Counter Tops And Surface Areas										
2	Wipe Down The Walls Wherever There Are Spills And Splashes										
3	Disinfect Touch Points, Light Switches And Other Switches										
4	Clean And Disinfect All Doors, Handles And Doorknobs										
5	Clean And Dust Door Frames, Remember To Dust The Tops										
6	Dust Light Fixtures With A Duster Or A Microfibre Cloth										
7	Wall Mirrors Cleaned With Glass Cleaner										
8	Clean Any Bathroom Glasses And Cups										
9	Clean And Sanitize Any Chairs And Seats										
10	Empty The Waste Basket And Recycling Bin										
11	Clean And Disinfectant The Waste Bin And Recycling Bin										
12	Clean And Wipe Down Windowsills										
13	Spray Air Freshener This Keeps The Room Smelling Fresh										
14	Air/Odour Control Systems Are Filled And Operating Correctly										
15	Clean Skirting Boards/Baseboards And Corners										
16	Vacuum And Hoover Bath Mats, Shower Mats And Rugs										
17	Replace Bath Mats, Shower Mats And Rugs With Clean Ones										
18	Steam Clean Carpets And Rugs										
19	Hand Towels Replaced With Fresh Clean Ones										
20	Bath Towels Replaced With Fresh Clean Ones										
21	Face Towels Replaced With Fresh Clean Ones										
22	Electric Hand Dryers Cleaned, Disinfected & Operating Correctly										
23	Soap Dispensers, Sanitizers And Hand Gels Are Refilled										
24	Clean & Check Contents Of Medicine Trolleys & Cupboards										
25	Clean And Disinfect Any Handrails										
26	Sinks, Taps And Fixtures Cleaned And Disinfected										
27	Clean And Disinfect Cabinets And Units										
28	Feminine Hygiene Dispensers Re-Stocked										
29	Feminine Hygiene Bins/Containers Emptied And Cleared										

Care Home Cleaning Tasks - Toilet & Restroom	M	T	W	T	F	S	S	Cleaned By	Checked By	Date/Time
Clean & Vacuum Central Heating Units (Backs Of Radiators)										
Wash And Clean Ceiling Light Covers										
Toilet Roll Holders And Toilet Rolls Re-Stocked										
Toilet Roll Holders Cleaned And Disinfected										
Clean Inside The Toilets And Urinals With Disinfectant										
Toilet Seats Cleaned And Disinfected										
Clean Top Of Toilets Tanks, The Bases And Behind Toilets										
Urinal Handles Cleaned And Disinfected										
Urinal Screens Cleaned, Disinfected And Blocks Replaced										
Paper Dispensers And Paper Towel Rolls Re-Stocked										
Paper Dispensers And Paper Towel Roll Cleaned & Disinfected										
The Floors Are Swept And Free From Debris And Litter										
Floors Mopped Clean With Cleaning Or Disinfecting Solution										
Put Up Or Place Wet Floor Signs After Mopping Floors										
Showers And Shower Heads, Cleaned And Disinfected										
Soak Shower Heads										
Clean And Disinfect Glass Shower Doors/Outer Doors										
Clean Soap Scum From Shower Walls										
Clean Blinds (Dust The Blinds With A Damp Microfibre Cloth)										
Clean Curtains (Vacuum On A Low Setting Or Wash If Possible)										
Dust And Wash Radiator Covers										
Clean And Disinfect Commodes Between Each Use										
Clean And Disinfect Shower Chairs Between Each Use										
Bath Hoists Cleaned And Disinfected Between Each Use										
Scrub Tub/Bath, Polish Facets And Taps, Clean & Disinfected										
Toothbrush Holders And Soap Holders Cleaned										
Re-Place Shower Curtains With Clean Fresh Ones										
Wash And Clean Air Vents										
Thoroughly Clean Grout And Tiles										
Disinfect And Clean All The Walls From Top To Bottom										
Wash And Clean Windows (Inside And Outside)										
Unclog The Drains (Sink, Bath And Shower)										
Pour Drain Cleaner Down Sink, Shower & Bath Drains										
Floor Drains And Drain Covers Are Open And Free Of Debris										
Hair Dryers Cleaned And Disinfected And Operating Correctly										
Light Bulbs Checked And None Functioning Bulbs Replaced										
Check Hardware, Door Stops And Lock Mechanisms										

CARE HOME BEDROOM CLEANING *Checklist*

Building	Location	Room Number	Area

Start Date & Time	Finnish Date & Time	Name	Signature

	Care Home Cleaning Tasks - Bedrooms	M	T	W	T	F	S	S	Cleaned By	Checked By	Date/Tim
1	Clean And Sanitize All The Desks And Tables										
2	Clean And Sanitize All The Counter Tops And Surface Areas										
3	Wipe Down The Walls Wherever There Are Spills And Splashes										
4	Disinfect Touch Points, Light Switches And Other Switches										
5	Clean And Disinfect All Doors, Handles And Doorknobs										
6	Clean And Dust Door Frames, Remember To Dust The Tops										
7	Dust Light Fixtures With A Duster Or A Microfibre Cloth										
8	Clean & Wipe Mirrors Remove Fingerprints, Smears & Dirt										
9	Clean And Dust Bedside Cabinets										
10	Clean And Sanitize Over Chair Tables										
11	Clean And Sanitize Over Bed Tables										
12	Clean And Check Bed Frames										
13	Mattresses Hoovered And Cleaned With Disinfectant										
14	Clean And Polish Bookshelves, Remember To Dust The Top										
15	Remove, Wash And Clean Any Dirty Cups Or Glasses										
16	Remove, Wash And Clean Any Dirty Plates, Bowels Or Cutlery										
17	Clean And Sanitize Any Chairs And Seats										
18	Water Jug (Washed Thoroughly Each Day & Re-Filled)										
19	Water Any Plants And Flowers										
20	Dust Plant Leafs (A Healthy Plant Needs To Be Clear Of Dust)										
21	Empty The Waste Basket And Recycling Bin										
22	Clean And Disinfectant The Waste Bin And Recycling Bin										
23	Clean And Wipe Down Windowsills										
24	Spray Air Freshener This Keeps The Room Smelling Fresh										
25	Clean And Disinfect Cabinets And Units										
26	Clean And Sanitize Desk Accessories										
27	Replace Dirty Linen And Move To Laundry Room										
28	Polish Any Wooden Furniture And Hardwood Surfaces										
29	Clean Skirting Boards/Baseboards And Corners										

Care Home Cleaning Tasks - Bedrooms Continued	M	T	W	T	F	S	S	Cleaned By	Checked By	Date/Time
Dust Television, Top Sides And Back, TV Unit And TV Stand										
Clean TV Screen With Soft Damp Cloth (Use Water/Cleaner)										
Vacuum/Hoover Between Bedroom Furniture And The Walls										
Clean And Sanitize Resident's Personal Wheelchair										
Check For Broken Wheelchairs, Frames and Wheels										
Vacuum Under Furniture, Beds, Sofas and Dressers										
Vacuum And Hoover The Carpets, Mats And Rugs										
Vacuum Furnishings, Cushions, Chairs, Sofas And Couches										
Steam Clean Carpets And Rugs										
Dust And Clean Any Picture Frames And Photo Frames										
Ledges, Flat Surfaces And The Tops Of Wardrobes Dusted										
Clean & Check Contents Of Medicine Trolleys & Cupboards										
Clean And Sanitize Mobile Phone, Phone Case And Screen										
Clean & Vacuum The Desk Chair, Legs And Chair Wheels										
Wash And Clean Air Vents										
Dust Ceiling Fan Blades With Duster Or A Microfibre Cloth										
Wash And Clean Windows (Inside And Outside)										
Dust And Clean The Walls From Top To Bottom										
Clean Blinds (Dust The Blinds With A Damp Microfibre Cloth)										
Clean Curtains (Vacuum On A Low Setting Or Wash If Possible)										
Dust And Wash Radiator Covers										
Wash And Clean Ceiling Light Covers										
Clean & Vacuum Central Heating Units (Backs Of Radiators)										
Clean And Disinfect Any Handrails										
Hand Towels Replaced With Fresh Clean Ones										
Sink Wall Mirror Cleaned With Glass Cleaner										
Sinks, Taps And Fixtures Cleaned And Disinfected										
Pour Drain Cleaner Down Sink Drains										
Check For Broken Furniture (Report/Schedule Maintenance)										
Light Bulbs Checked And None Functioning Bulbs Replaced										
Check Hardware, Door Stops And Lock Mechanisms										
Fire Exit Lights And Emergency Lights Checked & Functioning										
Test Carbon Monoxide Alarm And Replace Batteries If Required										
Test Smoke Detector Alarm And Replace Batteries If Required										
Paper Dispensers And Paper Towel Rolls Re-Stocked										
Soap Dispensers, Hand Sanitizers And Hand Gels Are Refilled										
Face Masks, Protective Gloves And Face Shields Re-Stocked										

CARE HOME COMMUNAL AREA CLEANING *Checklist*

Building	Location	Room Number	Area

Start Date & Time	Finnish Date & Time	Name	Signature

	Care Home Cleaning Tasks - Communal Area	M	T	W	T	F	S	S	Cleaned By	Checked By	Date/Tim
1	Clean And Sanitize All The Desks And Tables										
2	Clean And Sanitize All The Counter Tops And Surface Areas										
3	Wipe Down The Walls Wherever There Are Spills And Splashes										
4	Disinfect Touch Points, Light Switches And Other Switches										
5	Clean And Disinfect All Doors, Handles And Doorknobs										
6	Clean And Dust Door Frames, Remember To Dust The Tops										
7	Dust Light Fixtures & Shades With A Duster Or A Microfibre Cloth										
8	Clean And Wipe Mirrors Remove Fingerprints, Smears & Dirt										
9	Clean And Sanitize Over Chair Tables										
10	Clean And Polish Bookshelves, Remember To Dust The Top										
11	Remove, Wash And Clean Any Dirty Cups Or Glasses										
12	Remove, Wash And Clean Any Dirty Plates, Bowels Or Cutlery										
13	Clean And Sanitize Any Chairs, Seats And Benches										
14	Water Jugs (Washed Thoroughly Each Day & Re-Filled)										
15	Water Any Plants And Flowers										
16	Dust Plant Leafs (A Healthy Plant Needs To Be Clear Of Dust)										
17	Empty The Waste Baskets And Recycling Bins										
18	Clean And Disinfectant The Waste Bins And Recycling Bins										
19	Clean And Wipe Down Windowsills										
20	Spray Air Freshener This Keeps The Room Smelling Fresh										
21	Clean And Disinfect Cabinets And Units										
22	Clean And Sanitize Desk Accessories										
23	Replace Dirty Table Linen And Move To Laundry Room										
24	Polish Any Wooden Furniture And Hardwood Surfaces										
25	Clean Skirting Boards/Baseboards And Corners										
26	Clean And Polish Fireplace Mantelpiece And Surrounds										
27	Wipe Down Equipment & Sanitize Tea And Coffee Making Facilities										
28	Clean And Sanitize Telephones, Cords/Leads & All Touch Points										
29	Clean And Sanitize Walking Sticks And Any Other Walking Aids										

Care Home Cleaning Tasks - Communal Area	M	T	W	T	F	S	S	Cleaned By	Checked By	Date/Time
Dust Television, Top Sides And Back, TV Unit And TV Stand										
Clean TV Screen With Soft Damp Cloth (Use Water/Cleaner)										
Vacuum/Hoover Between Furniture And The Walls										
Clean And Sanitize All Wheelchairs										
Check For Broken Wheelchairs, Frames and Wheels										
Vacuum Under Furniture, Units, Tables And Cabinets										
Vacuum And Hoover The Carpets, Mats And Rugs										
Vacuum Furnishings, Cushions, Chairs, Sofas And Couches										
Steam Clean Carpets And Rugs										
Dust And Clean Any Picture Frames And Wall Art										
Clean & Check Contents Of Medicine Trolleys & Cupboards										
Clean & Vacuum The Desk Chair, Legs And Chair Wheels										
Wash And Clean Air Vents										
Dust Ceiling Fan Blades With Duster Or A Microfibre Cloth										
Wash And Clean Windows (Inside And Outside)										
Dust And Clean The Walls From Top To Bottom										
Clean Blinds (Dust The Blinds With A Damp Microfibre Cloth)										
Clean Curtains (Vacuum On A Low Setting Or Wash If Possible)										
Dust And Wash Radiator Covers										
Wash And Clean Ceiling Light Covers										
Clean & Vacuum Central Heating Units (Backs Of Radiators)										
Clean And Disinfect Any Handrails										
Clean And Sanitize Computer, Keyboard And Computer Mice										
Clean And Sanitize iPads, Tablets, Laptops & Mobile Phones										
Floors Mopped Clean With Cleaning Or Disinfecting Solution										
The Floors Are Swept And Free From Debris And Litter										
Clean Sliding Doors and Room Partitions										
Throw Away Outdated Newspapers, Magazines, Papers										
Check For Broken Furniture (Report/Schedule Maintenance)										
Light Bulbs Checked And None Functioning Bulbs Replaced										
Check Hardware, Door Stops And Lock Mechanisms										
Fire Exit Lights And Emergency Lights Checked & Functioning										
Test Carbon Monoxide Alarm And Replace Batteries If Required										
Test Smoke Detector Alarm And Replace Batteries If Required										
Paper Dispensers And Paper Towel Rolls Re-Stocked										
Soap Dispensers, Hand Sanitizers And Hand Gels Are Refilled										
Face Masks, Protective Gloves And Face Shields Re-Stocked										

CARE HOME TOILET & RESTROOM CLEANING *Checklist*

Building	Location	Room Number	Area

Start Date & Time	Finnish Date & Time	Name	Signature

	Care Home Cleaning Tasks - Toilet & Restroom	M	T	W	T	F	S	S	Cleaned By	Checked By	Date/Time
1	Clean And Sanitize All The Counter Tops And Surface Areas										
2	Wipe Down The Walls Wherever There Are Spills And Splashes										
3	Disinfect Touch Points, Light Switches And Other Switches										
4	Clean And Disinfect All Doors, Handles And Doorknobs										
5	Clean And Dust Door Frames, Remember To Dust The Tops										
6	Dust Light Fixtures With A Duster Or A Microfibre Cloth										
7	Wall Mirrors Cleaned With Glass Cleaner										
8	Clean Any Bathroom Glasses And Cups										
9	Clean And Sanitize Any Chairs And Seats										
10	Empty The Waste Basket And Recycling Bin										
11	Clean And Disinfectant The Waste Bin And Recycling Bin										
12	Clean And Wipe Down Windowsills										
13	Spray Air Freshener This Keeps The Room Smelling Fresh										
14	Air/Odour Control Systems Are Filled And Operating Correctly										
15	Clean Skirting Boards/Baseboards And Corners										
16	Vacuum And Hoover Bath Mats, Shower Mats And Rugs										
17	Replace Bath Mats, Shower Mats And Rugs With Clean Ones										
18	Steam Clean Carpets And Rugs										
19	Hand Towels Replaced With Fresh Clean Ones										
20	Bath Towels Replaced With Fresh Clean Ones										
21	Face Towels Replaced With Fresh Clean Ones										
22	Electric Hand Dryers Cleaned, Disinfected & Operating Correctly										
23	Soap Dispensers, Sanitizers And Hand Gels Are Refilled										
24	Clean & Check Contents Of Medicine Trolleys & Cupboards										
25	Clean And Disinfect Any Handrails										
26	Sinks, Taps And Fixtures Cleaned And Disinfected										
27	Clean And Disinfect Cabinets And Units										
28	Feminine Hygiene Dispensers Re-Stocked										
29	Feminine Hygiene Bins/Containers Emptied And Cleared										

Care Home Cleaning Tasks - Toilet & Restroom	M	T	W	T	F	S	S	Cleaned By	Checked By	Date/Time
Clean & Vacuum Central Heating Units (Backs Of Radiators)										
Wash And Clean Ceiling Light Covers										
Toilet Roll Holders And Toilet Rolls Re-Stocked										
Toilet Roll Holders Cleaned And Disinfected										
Clean Inside The Toilets And Urinals With Disinfectant										
Toilet Seats Cleaned And Disinfected										
Clean Top Of Toilets Tanks, The Bases And Behind Toilets										
Urinal Handles Cleaned And Disinfected										
Urinal Screens Cleaned, Disinfected And Blocks Replaced										
Paper Dispensers And Paper Towel Rolls Re-Stocked										
Paper Dispensers And Paper Towel Roll Cleaned & Disinfected										
The Floors Are Swept And Free From Debris And Litter										
Floors Mopped Clean With Cleaning Or Disinfecting Solution										
Put Up Or Place Wet Floor Signs After Mopping Floors										
Showers And Shower Heads, Cleaned And Disinfected										
Soak Shower Heads										
Clean And Disinfect Glass Shower Doors/Outer Doors										
Clean Soap Scum From Shower Walls										
Clean Blinds (Dust The Blinds With A Damp Microfibre Cloth)										
Clean Curtains (Vacuum On A Low Setting Or Wash If Possible)										
Dust And Wash Radiator Covers										
Clean And Disinfect Commodes Between Each Use										
Clean And Disinfect Shower Chairs Between Each Use										
Bath Hoists Cleaned And Disinfected Between Each Use										
Scrub Tub/Bath, Polish Facets And Taps, Clean & Disinfected										
Toothbrush Holders And Soap Holders Cleaned										
Re-Place Shower Curtains With Clean Fresh Ones										
Wash And Clean Air Vents										
Thoroughly Clean Grout And Tiles										
Disinfect And Clean All The Walls From Top To Bottom										
Wash And Clean Windows (Inside And Outside)										
Unclog The Drains (Sink, Bath And Shower)										
Pour Drain Cleaner Down Sink, Shower & Bath Drains										
Floor Drains And Drain Covers Are Open And Free Of Debris										
Hair Dryers Cleaned And Disinfected And Operating Correctly										
Light Bulbs Checked And None Functioning Bulbs Replaced										
Check Hardware, Door Stops And Lock Mechanisms										

CARE HOME BEDROOM CLEANING *Checklist*

Building	Location	Room Number	Area

Start Date & Time	Finnish Date & Time	Name	Signature

	Care Home Cleaning Tasks - Bedrooms	M	T	W	T	F	S	S	Cleaned By	Checked By	Date/Tim
1	Clean And Sanitize All The Desks And Tables										
2	Clean And Sanitize All The Counter Tops And Surface Areas										
3	Wipe Down The Walls Wherever There Are Spills And Splashes										
4	Disinfect Touch Points, Light Switches And Other Switches										
5	Clean And Disinfect All Doors, Handles And Doorknobs										
6	Clean And Dust Door Frames, Remember To Dust The Tops										
7	Dust Light Fixtures With A Duster Or A Microfibre Cloth										
8	Clean & Wipe Mirrors Remove Fingerprints, Smears & Dirt										
9	Clean And Dust Bedside Cabinets										
10	Clean And Sanitize Over Chair Tables										
11	Clean And Sanitize Over Bed Tables										
12	Clean And Check Bed Frames										
13	Mattresses Hoovered And Cleaned With Disinfectant										
14	Clean And Polish Bookshelves, Remember To Dust The Top										
15	Remove, Wash And Clean Any Dirty Cups Or Glasses										
16	Remove, Wash And Clean Any Dirty Plates, Bowels Or Cutlery										
17	Clean And Sanitize Any Chairs And Seats										
18	Water Jug (Washed Thoroughly Each Day & Re-Filled)										
19	Water Any Plants And Flowers										
20	Dust Plant Leafs (A Healthy Plant Needs To Be Clear Of Dust)										
21	Empty The Waste Basket And Recycling Bin										
22	Clean And Disinfectant The Waste Bin And Recycling Bin										
23	Clean And Wipe Down Windowsills										
24	Spray Air Freshener This Keeps The Room Smelling Fresh										
25	Clean And Disinfect Cabinets And Units										
26	Clean And Sanitize Desk Accessories										
27	Replace Dirty Linen And Move To Laundry Room										
28	Polish Any Wooden Furniture And Hardwood Surfaces										
29	Clean Skirting Boards/Baseboards And Corners										

Care Home Cleaning Tasks - Bedrooms Continued	M	T	W	T	F	S	S	Cleaned By	Checked By	Date/Time
Dust Television, Top Sides And Back, TV Unit And TV Stand										
Clean TV Screen With Soft Damp Cloth (Use Water/Cleaner)										
Vacuum/Hoover Between Bedroom Furniture And The Walls										
Clean And Sanitize Resident's Personal Wheelchair										
Check For Broken Wheelchairs, Frames and Wheels										
Vacuum Under Furniture, Beds, Sofas and Dressers										
Vacuum And Hoover The Carpets, Mats And Rugs										
Vacuum Furnishings, Cushions, Chairs, Sofas And Couches										
Steam Clean Carpets And Rugs										
Dust And Clean Any Picture Frames And Photo Frames										
Ledges, Flat Surfaces And The Tops Of Wardrobes Dusted										
Clean & Check Contents Of Medicine Trolleys & Cupboards										
Clean And Sanitize Mobile Phone, Phone Case And Screen										
Clean & Vacuum The Desk Chair, Legs And Chair Wheels										
Wash And Clean Air Vents										
Dust Ceiling Fan Blades With Duster Or A Microfibre Cloth										
Wash And Clean Windows (Inside And Outside)										
Dust And Clean The Walls From Top To Bottom										
Clean Blinds (Dust The Blinds With A Damp Microfibre Cloth)										
Clean Curtains (Vacuum On A Low Setting Or Wash If Possible)										
Dust And Wash Radiator Covers										
Wash And Clean Ceiling Light Covers										
Clean & Vacuum Central Heating Units (Backs Of Radiators)										
Clean And Disinfect Any Handrails										
Hand Towels Replaced With Fresh Clean Ones										
Sink Wall Mirror Cleaned With Glass Cleaner										
Sinks, Taps And Fixtures Cleaned And Disinfected										
Pour Drain Cleaner Down Sink Drains										
Check For Broken Furniture (Report/Schedule Maintenance)										
Light Bulbs Checked And None Functioning Bulbs Replaced										
Check Hardware, Door Stops And Lock Mechanisms										
Fire Exit Lights And Emergency Lights Checked & Functioning										
Test Carbon Monoxide Alarm And Replace Batteries If Required										
Test Smoke Detector Alarm And Replace Batteries If Required										
Paper Dispensers And Paper Towel Rolls Re-Stocked										
Soap Dispensers, Hand Sanitizers And Hand Gels Are Refilled										
Face Masks, Protective Gloves And Face Shields Re-Stocked										

CARE HOME COMMUNAL AREA CLEANING *Checklist*

Building	Location	Room Number	Area

Start Date & Time	Finnish Date & Time	Name	Signature

	Care Home Cleaning Tasks - Communal Area	M	T	W	T	F	S	S	Cleaned By	Checked By	Date/Tim
1	Clean And Sanitize All The Desks And Tables										
2	Clean And Sanitize All The Counter Tops And Surface Areas										
3	Wipe Down The Walls Wherever There Are Spills And Splashes										
4	Disinfect Touch Points, Light Switches And Other Switches										
5	Clean And Disinfect All Doors, Handles And Doorknobs										
6	Clean And Dust Door Frames, Remember To Dust The Tops										
7	Dust Light Fixtures & Shades With A Duster Or A Microfibre Cloth										
8	Clean And Wipe Mirrors Remove Fingerprints, Smears & Dirt										
9	Clean And Sanitize Over Chair Tables										
10	Clean And Polish Bookshelves, Remember To Dust The Top										
11	Remove, Wash And Clean Any Dirty Cups Or Glasses										
12	Remove, Wash And Clean Any Dirty Plates, Bowels Or Cutlery										
13	Clean And Sanitize Any Chairs, Seats And Benches										
14	Water Jugs (Washed Thoroughly Each Day & Re-Filled)										
15	Water Any Plants And Flowers										
16	Dust Plant Leafs (A Healthy Plant Needs To Be Clear Of Dust)										
17	Empty The Waste Baskets And Recycling Bins										
18	Clean And Disinfectant The Waste Bins And Recycling Bins										
19	Clean And Wipe Down Windowsills										
20	Spray Air Freshener This Keeps The Room Smelling Fresh										
21	Clean And Disinfect Cabinets And Units										
22	Clean And Sanitize Desk Accessories										
23	Replace Dirty Table Linen And Move To Laundry Room										
24	Polish Any Wooden Furniture And Hardwood Surfaces										
25	Clean Skirting Boards/Baseboards And Corners										
26	Clean And Polish Fireplace Mantelpiece And Surrounds										
27	Wipe Down Equipment & Sanitize Tea And Coffee Making Facilities										
28	Clean And Sanitize Telephones, Cords/Leads & All Touch Points										
29	Clean And Sanitize Walking Sticks And Any Other Walking Aids										

Care Home Cleaning Tasks - Communal Area	M	T	W	T	F	S	S	Cleaned By	Checked By	Date/Time
Dust Television, Top Sides And Back, TV Unit And TV Stand										
Clean TV Screen With Soft Damp Cloth (Use Water/Cleaner)										
Vacuum/Hoover Between Furniture And The Walls										
Clean And Sanitize All Wheelchairs										
Check For Broken Wheelchairs, Frames and Wheels										
Vacuum Under Furniture, Units, Tables And Cabinets										
Vacuum And Hoover The Carpets, Mats And Rugs										
Vacuum Furnishings, Cushions, Chairs, Sofas And Couches										
Steam Clean Carpets And Rugs										
Dust And Clean Any Picture Frames And Wall Art										
Clean & Check Contents Of Medicine Trolleys & Cupboards										
Clean & Vacuum The Desk Chair, Legs And Chair Wheels										
Wash And Clean Air Vents										
Dust Ceiling Fan Blades With Duster Or A Microfibre Cloth										
Wash And Clean Windows (Inside And Outside)										
Dust And Clean The Walls From Top To Bottom										
Clean Blinds (Dust The Blinds With A Damp Microfibre Cloth)										
Clean Curtains (Vacuum On A Low Setting Or Wash If Possible)										
Dust And Wash Radiator Covers										
Wash And Clean Ceiling Light Covers										
Clean & Vacuum Central Heating Units (Backs Of Radiators)										
Clean And Disinfect Any Handrails										
Clean And Sanitize Computer, Keyboard And Computer Mice										
Clean And Sanitize iPads, Tablets, Laptops & Mobile Phones										
Floors Mopped Clean With Cleaning Or Disinfecting Solution										
The Floors Are Swept And Free From Debris And Litter										
Clean Sliding Doors and Room Partitions										
Throw Away Outdated Newspapers, Magazines, Papers										
Check For Broken Furniture (Report/Schedule Maintenance)										
Light Bulbs Checked And None Functioning Bulbs Replaced										
Check Hardware, Door Stops And Lock Mechanisms										
Fire Exit Lights And Emergency Lights Checked & Functioning										
Test Carbon Monoxide Alarm And Replace Batteries If Required										
Test Smoke Detector Alarm And Replace Batteries If Required										
Paper Dispensers And Paper Towel Rolls Re-Stocked										
Soap Dispensers, Hand Sanitizers And Hand Gels Are Refilled										
Face Masks, Protective Gloves And Face Shields Re-Stocked										

CARE HOME TOILET & RESTROOM CLEANING *Checklist*

Building	Location	Room Number	Area

Start Date & Time	Finnish Date & Time	Name	Signature

	Care Home Cleaning Tasks - Toilet & Restroom	M	T	W	T	F	S	S	Cleaned By	Checked By	Date/Tim
1	Clean And Sanitize All The Counter Tops And Surface Areas										
2	Wipe Down The Walls Wherever There Are Spills And Splashes										
3	Disinfect Touch Points, Light Switches And Other Switches										
4	Clean And Disinfect All Doors, Handles And Doorknobs										
5	Clean And Dust Door Frames, Remember To Dust The Tops										
6	Dust Light Fixtures With A Duster Or A Microfibre Cloth										
7	Wall Mirrors Cleaned With Glass Cleaner										
8	Clean Any Bathroom Glasses And Cups										
9	Clean And Sanitize Any Chairs And Seats										
10	Empty The Waste Basket And Recycling Bin										
11	Clean And Disinfectant The Waste Bin And Recycling Bin										
12	Clean And Wipe Down Windowsills										
13	Spray Air Freshener This Keeps The Room Smelling Fresh										
14	Air/Odour Control Systems Are Filled And Operating Correctly										
15	Clean Skirting Boards/Baseboards And Corners										
16	Vacuum And Hoover Bath Mats, Shower Mats And Rugs										
17	Replace Bath Mats, Shower Mats And Rugs With Clean Ones										
18	Steam Clean Carpets And Rugs										
19	Hand Towels Replaced With Fresh Clean Ones										
20	Bath Towels Replaced With Fresh Clean Ones										
21	Face Towels Replaced With Fresh Clean Ones										
22	Electric Hand Dryers Cleaned, Disinfected & Operating Correctly										
23	Soap Dispensers, Sanitizers And Hand Gels Are Refilled										
24	Clean & Check Contents Of Medicine Trolleys & Cupboards										
25	Clean And Disinfect Any Handrails										
26	Sinks, Taps And Fixtures Cleaned And Disinfected										
27	Clean And Disinfect Cabinets And Units										
28	Feminine Hygiene Dispensers Re-Stocked										
29	Feminine Hygiene Bins/Containers Emptied And Cleared										

Care Home Cleaning Tasks - Toilet & Restroom	M	T	W	T	F	S	S	Cleaned By	Checked By	Date/Time
Clean & Vacuum Central Heating Units (Backs Of Radiators)										
Wash And Clean Ceiling Light Covers										
Toilet Roll Holders And Toilet Rolls Re-Stocked										
Toilet Roll Holders Cleaned And Disinfected										
Clean Inside The Toilets And Urinals With Disinfectant										
Toilet Seats Cleaned And Disinfected										
Clean Top Of Toilets Tanks, The Bases And Behind Toilets										
Urinal Handles Cleaned And Disinfected										
Urinal Screens Cleaned, Disinfected And Blocks Replaced										
Paper Dispensers And Paper Towel Rolls Re-Stocked										
Paper Dispensers And Paper Towel Roll Cleaned & Disinfected										
The Floors Are Swept And Free From Debris And Litter										
Floors Mopped Clean With Cleaning Or Disinfecting Solution										
Put Up Or Place Wet Floor Signs After Mopping Floors										
Showers And Shower Heads, Cleaned And Disinfected										
Soak Shower Heads										
Clean And Disinfect Glass Shower Doors/Outer Doors										
Clean Soap Scum From Shower Walls										
Clean Blinds (Dust The Blinds With A Damp Microfibre Cloth)										
Clean Curtains (Vacuum On A Low Setting Or Wash If Possible)										
Dust And Wash Radiator Covers										
Clean And Disinfect Commodes Between Each Use										
Clean And Disinfect Shower Chairs Between Each Use										
Bath Hoists Cleaned And Disinfected Between Each Use										
Scrub Tub/Bath, Polish Facets And Taps, Clean & Disinfected										
Toothbrush Holders And Soap Holders Cleaned										
Re-Place Shower Curtains With Clean Fresh Ones										
Wash And Clean Air Vents										
Thoroughly Clean Grout And Tiles										
Disinfect And Clean All The Walls From Top To Bottom										
Wash And Clean Windows (Inside And Outside)										
Unclog The Drains (Sink, Bath And Shower)										
Pour Drain Cleaner Down Sink, Shower & Bath Drains										
Floor Drains And Drain Covers Are Open And Free Of Debris										
Hair Dryers Cleaned And Disinfected And Operating Correctly										
Light Bulbs Checked And None Functioning Bulbs Replaced										
Check Hardware, Door Stops And Lock Mechanisms										

CARE HOME BEDROOM CLEANING *Checklist*

Building	Location	Room Number	Area

Start Date & Time	Finnish Date & Time	Name	Signature

	Care Home Cleaning Tasks - Bedrooms	M	T	W	T	F	S	S	Cleaned By	Checked By	Date/Tim
1	Clean And Sanitize All The Desks And Tables										
2	Clean And Sanitize All The Counter Tops And Surface Areas										
3	Wipe Down The Walls Wherever There Are Spills And Splashes										
4	Disinfect Touch Points, Light Switches And Other Switches										
5	Clean And Disinfect All Doors, Handles And Doorknobs										
6	Clean And Dust Door Frames, Remember To Dust The Tops										
7	Dust Light Fixtures With A Duster Or A Microfibre Cloth										
8	Clean & Wipe Mirrors Remove Fingerprints, Smears & Dirt										
9	Clean And Dust Bedside Cabinets										
10	Clean And Sanitize Over Chair Tables										
11	Clean And Sanitize Over Bed Tables										
12	Clean And Check Bed Frames										
13	Mattresses Hoovered And Cleaned With Disinfectant										
14	Clean And Polish Bookshelves, Remember To Dust The Top										
15	Remove, Wash And Clean Any Dirty Cups Or Glasses										
16	Remove, Wash And Clean Any Dirty Plates, Bowels Or Cutlery										
17	Clean And Sanitize Any Chairs And Seats										
18	Water Jug (Washed Thoroughly Each Day & Re-Filled)										
19	Water Any Plants And Flowers										
20	Dust Plant Leafs (A Healthy Plant Needs To Be Clear Of Dust)										
21	Empty The Waste Basket And Recycling Bin										
22	Clean And Disinfectant The Waste Bin And Recycling Bin										
23	Clean And Wipe Down Windowsills										
24	Spray Air Freshener This Keeps The Room Smelling Fresh										
25	Clean And Disinfect Cabinets And Units										
26	Clean And Sanitize Desk Accessories										
27	Replace Dirty Linen And Move To Laundry Room										
28	Polish Any Wooden Furniture And Hardwood Surfaces										
29	Clean Skirting Boards/Baseboards And Corners										

Care Home Cleaning Tasks - Bedrooms Continued	M	T	W	T	F	S	S	Cleaned By	Checked By	Date/Time
Dust Television, Top Sides And Back, TV Unit And TV Stand										
Clean TV Screen With Soft Damp Cloth (Use Water/Cleaner)										
Vacuum/Hoover Between Bedroom Furniture And The Walls										
Clean And Sanitize Resident's Personal Wheelchair										
Check For Broken Wheelchairs, Frames and Wheels										
Vacuum Under Furniture, Beds, Sofas and Dressers										
Vacuum And Hoover The Carpets, Mats And Rugs										
Vacuum Furnishings, Cushions, Chairs, Sofas And Couches										
Steam Clean Carpets And Rugs										
Dust And Clean Any Picture Frames And Photo Frames										
Ledges, Flat Surfaces And The Tops Of Wardrobes Dusted										
Clean & Check Contents Of Medicine Trolleys & Cupboards										
Clean And Sanitize Mobile Phone, Phone Case And Screen										
Clean & Vacuum The Desk Chair, Legs And Chair Wheels										
Wash And Clean Air Vents										
Dust Ceiling Fan Blades With Duster Or A Microfibre Cloth										
Wash And Clean Windows (Inside And Outside)										
Dust And Clean The Walls From Top To Bottom										
Clean Blinds (Dust The Blinds With A Damp Microfibre Cloth)										
Clean Curtains (Vacuum On A Low Setting Or Wash If Possible)										
Dust And Wash Radiator Covers										
Wash And Clean Ceiling Light Covers										
Clean & Vacuum Central Heating Units (Backs Of Radiators)										
Clean And Disinfect Any Handrails										
Hand Towels Replaced With Fresh Clean Ones										
Sink Wall Mirror Cleaned With Glass Cleaner										
Sinks, Taps And Fixtures Cleaned And Disinfected										
Pour Drain Cleaner Down Sink Drains										
Check For Broken Furniture (Report/Schedule Maintenance)										
Light Bulbs Checked And None Functioning Bulbs Replaced										
Check Hardware, Door Stops And Lock Mechanisms										
Fire Exit Lights And Emergency Lights Checked & Functioning										
Test Carbon Monoxide Alarm And Replace Batteries If Required										
Test Smoke Detector Alarm And Replace Batteries If Required										
Paper Dispensers And Paper Towel Rolls Re-Stocked										
Soap Dispensers, Hand Sanitizers And Hand Gels Are Refilled										
Face Masks, Protective Gloves And Face Shields Re-Stocked										

CARE HOME COMMUNAL AREA CLEANING *Checklist*

Building	Location	Room Number	Area

Start Date & Time	Finnish Date & Time	Name	Signature

	Care Home Cleaning Tasks - Communal Area	M	T	W	T	F	S	S	Cleaned By	Checked By	Date/Tim
1	Clean And Sanitize All The Desks And Tables										
2	Clean And Sanitize All The Counter Tops And Surface Areas										
3	Wipe Down The Walls Wherever There Are Spills And Splashes										
4	Disinfect Touch Points, Light Switches And Other Switches										
5	Clean And Disinfect All Doors, Handles And Doorknobs										
6	Clean And Dust Door Frames, Remember To Dust The Tops										
7	Dust Light Fixtures & Shades With A Duster Or A Microfibre Cloth										
8	Clean And Wipe Mirrors Remove Fingerprints, Smears & Dirt										
9	Clean And Sanitize Over Chair Tables										
10	Clean And Polish Bookshelves, Remember To Dust The Top										
11	Remove, Wash And Clean Any Dirty Cups Or Glasses										
12	Remove, Wash And Clean Any Dirty Plates, Bowels Or Cutlery										
13	Clean And Sanitize Any Chairs, Seats And Benches										
14	Water Jugs (Washed Thoroughly Each Day & Re-Filled)										
15	Water Any Plants And Flowers										
16	Dust Plant Leafs (A Healthy Plant Needs To Be Clear Of Dust)										
17	Empty The Waste Baskets And Recycling Bins										
18	Clean And Disinfectant The Waste Bins And Recycling Bins										
19	Clean And Wipe Down Windowsills										
20	Spray Air Freshener This Keeps The Room Smelling Fresh										
21	Clean And Disinfect Cabinets And Units										
22	Clean And Sanitize Desk Accessories										
23	Replace Dirty Table Linen And Move To Laundry Room										
24	Polish Any Wooden Furniture And Hardwood Surfaces										
25	Clean Skirting Boards/Baseboards And Corners										
26	Clean And Polish Fireplace Mantelpiece And Surrounds										
27	Wipe Down Equipment & Sanitize Tea And Coffee Making Facilities										
28	Clean And Sanitize Telephones, Cords/Leads & All Touch Points										
29	Clean And Sanitize Walking Sticks And Any Other Walking Aids										

Care Home Cleaning Tasks - Communal Area	M	T	W	T	F	S	S	Cleaned By	Checked By	Date/Time
Dust Television, Top Sides And Back, TV Unit And TV Stand										
Clean TV Screen With Soft Damp Cloth (Use Water/Cleaner)										
Vacuum/Hoover Between Furniture And The Walls										
Clean And Sanitize All Wheelchairs										
Check For Broken Wheelchairs, Frames and Wheels										
Vacuum Under Furniture, Units, Tables And Cabinets										
Vacuum And Hoover The Carpets, Mats And Rugs										
Vacuum Furnishings, Cushions, Chairs, Sofas And Couches										
Steam Clean Carpets And Rugs										
Dust And Clean Any Picture Frames And Wall Art										
Clean & Check Contents Of Medicine Trolleys & Cupboards										
Clean & Vacuum The Desk Chair, Legs And Chair Wheels										
Wash And Clean Air Vents										
Dust Ceiling Fan Blades With Duster Or A Microfibre Cloth										
Wash And Clean Windows (Inside And Outside)										
Dust And Clean The Walls From Top To Bottom										
Clean Blinds (Dust The Blinds With A Damp Microfibre Cloth)										
Clean Curtains (Vacuum On A Low Setting Or Wash If Possible)										
Dust And Wash Radiator Covers										
Wash And Clean Ceiling Light Covers										
Clean & Vacuum Central Heating Units (Backs Of Radiators)										
Clean And Disinfect Any Handrails										
Clean And Sanitize Computer, Keyboard And Computer Mice										
Clean And Sanitize iPads, Tablets, Laptops & Mobile Phones										
Floors Mopped Clean With Cleaning Or Disinfecting Solution										
The Floors Are Swept And Free From Debris And Litter										
Clean Sliding Doors and Room Partitions										
Throw Away Outdated Newspapers, Magazines, Papers										
Check For Broken Furniture (Report/Schedule Maintenance)										
Light Bulbs Checked And None Functioning Bulbs Replaced										
Check Hardware, Door Stops And Lock Mechanisms										
Fire Exit Lights And Emergency Lights Checked & Functioning										
Test Carbon Monoxide Alarm And Replace Batteries If Required										
Test Smoke Detector Alarm And Replace Batteries If Required										
Paper Dispensers And Paper Towel Rolls Re-Stocked										
Soap Dispensers, Hand Sanitizers And Hand Gels Are Refilled										
Face Masks, Protective Gloves And Face Shields Re-Stocked										

CARE HOME TOILET & RESTROOM CLEANING *Checklist*

Building	Location	Room Number	Area

Start Date & Time	Finnish Date & Time	Name	Signature

	Care Home Cleaning Tasks - Toilet & Restroom	M	T	W	T	F	S	S	Cleaned By	Checked By	Date/Time
1	Clean And Sanitize All The Counter Tops And Surface Areas										
2	Wipe Down The Walls Wherever There Are Spills And Splashes										
3	Disinfect Touch Points, Light Switches And Other Switches										
4	Clean And Disinfect All Doors, Handles And Doorknobs										
5	Clean And Dust Door Frames, Remember To Dust The Tops										
6	Dust Light Fixtures With A Duster Or A Microfibre Cloth										
7	Wall Mirrors Cleaned With Glass Cleaner										
8	Clean Any Bathroom Glasses And Cups										
9	Clean And Sanitize Any Chairs And Seats										
10	Empty The Waste Basket And Recycling Bin										
11	Clean And Disinfectant The Waste Bin And Recycling Bin										
12	Clean And Wipe Down Windowsills										
13	Spray Air Freshener This Keeps The Room Smelling Fresh										
14	Air/Odour Control Systems Are Filled And Operating Correctly										
15	Clean Skirting Boards/Baseboards And Corners										
16	Vacuum And Hoover Bath Mats, Shower Mats And Rugs										
17	Replace Bath Mats, Shower Mats And Rugs With Clean Ones										
18	Steam Clean Carpets And Rugs										
19	Hand Towels Replaced With Fresh Clean Ones										
20	Bath Towels Replaced With Fresh Clean Ones										
21	Face Towels Replaced With Fresh Clean Ones										
22	Electric Hand Dryers Cleaned, Disinfected & Operating Correctly										
23	Soap Dispensers, Sanitizers And Hand Gels Are Refilled										
24	Clean & Check Contents Of Medicine Trolleys & Cupboards										
25	Clean And Disinfect Any Handrails										
26	Sinks, Taps And Fixtures Cleaned And Disinfected										
27	Clean And Disinfect Cabinets And Units										
28	Feminine Hygiene Dispensers Re-Stocked										
29	Feminine Hygiene Bins/Containers Emptied And Cleared										

Care Home Cleaning Tasks - Toilet & Restroom	M	T	W	T	F	S	S	Cleaned By	Checked By	Date/Time
Clean & Vacuum Central Heating Units (Backs Of Radiators)										
Wash And Clean Ceiling Light Covers										
Toilet Roll Holders And Toilet Rolls Re-Stocked										
Toilet Roll Holders Cleaned And Disinfected										
Clean Inside The Toilets And Urinals With Disinfectant										
Toilet Seats Cleaned And Disinfected										
Clean Top Of Toilets Tanks, The Bases And Behind Toilets										
Urinal Handles Cleaned And Disinfected										
Urinal Screens Cleaned, Disinfected And Blocks Replaced										
Paper Dispensers And Paper Towel Rolls Re-Stocked										
Paper Dispensers And Paper Towel Roll Cleaned & Disinfected										
The Floors Are Swept And Free From Debris And Litter										
Floors Mopped Clean With Cleaning Or Disinfecting Solution										
Put Up Or Place Wet Floor Signs After Mopping Floors										
Showers And Shower Heads, Cleaned And Disinfected										
Soak Shower Heads										
Clean And Disinfect Glass Shower Doors/Outer Doors										
Clean Soap Scum From Shower Walls										
Clean Blinds (Dust The Blinds With A Damp Microfibre Cloth)										
Clean Curtains (Vacuum On A Low Setting Or Wash If Possible)										
Dust And Wash Radiator Covers										
Clean And Disinfect Commodes Between Each Use										
Clean And Disinfect Shower Chairs Between Each Use										
Bath Hoists Cleaned And Disinfected Between Each Use										
Scrub Tub/Bath, Polish Facets And Taps, Clean & Disinfected										
Toothbrush Holders And Soap Holders Cleaned										
Re-Place Shower Curtains With Clean Fresh Ones										
Wash And Clean Air Vents										
Thoroughly Clean Grout And Tiles										
Disinfect And Clean All The Walls From Top To Bottom										
Wash And Clean Windows (Inside And Outside)										
Unclog The Drains (Sink, Bath And Shower)										
Pour Drain Cleaner Down Sink, Shower & Bath Drains										
Floor Drains And Drain Covers Are Open And Free Of Debris										
Hair Dryers Cleaned And Disinfected And Operating Correctly										
Light Bulbs Checked And None Functioning Bulbs Replaced										
Check Hardware, Door Stops And Lock Mechanisms										

CARE HOME BEDROOM CLEANING *Checklist*

Building	Location	Room Number	Area

Start Date & Time	Finnish Date & Time	Name	Signature

	Care Home Cleaning Tasks - Bedrooms	M	T	W	T	F	S	S	Cleaned By	Checked By	Date/Tim
1	Clean And Sanitize All The Desks And Tables										
2	Clean And Sanitize All The Counter Tops And Surface Areas										
3	Wipe Down The Walls Wherever There Are Spills And Splashes										
4	Disinfect Touch Points, Light Switches And Other Switches										
5	Clean And Disinfect All Doors, Handles And Doorknobs										
6	Clean And Dust Door Frames, Remember To Dust The Tops										
7	Dust Light Fixtures With A Duster Or A Microfibre Cloth										
8	Clean & Wipe Mirrors Remove Fingerprints, Smears & Dirt										
9	Clean And Dust Bedside Cabinets										
10	Clean And Sanitize Over Chair Tables										
11	Clean And Sanitize Over Bed Tables										
12	Clean And Check Bed Frames										
13	Mattresses Hoovered And Cleaned With Disinfectant										
14	Clean And Polish Bookshelves, Remember To Dust The Top										
15	Remove, Wash And Clean Any Dirty Cups Or Glasses										
16	Remove, Wash And Clean Any Dirty Plates, Bowels Or Cutlery										
17	Clean And Sanitize Any Chairs And Seats										
18	Water Jug (Washed Thoroughly Each Day & Re-Filled)										
19	Water Any Plants And Flowers										
20	Dust Plant Leafs (A Healthy Plant Needs To Be Clear Of Dust)										
21	Empty The Waste Basket And Recycling Bin										
22	Clean And Disinfectant The Waste Bin And Recycling Bin										
23	Clean And Wipe Down Windowsills										
24	Spray Air Freshener This Keeps The Room Smelling Fresh										
25	Clean And Disinfect Cabinets And Units										
26	Clean And Sanitize Desk Accessories										
27	Replace Dirty Linen And Move To Laundry Room										
28	Polish Any Wooden Furniture And Hardwood Surfaces										
29	Clean Skirting Boards/Baseboards And Corners										

Care Home Cleaning Tasks - Bedrooms Continued	M	T	W	T	F	S	S	Cleaned By	Checked By	Date/Time
Dust Television, Top Sides And Back, TV Unit And TV Stand										
Clean TV Screen With Soft Damp Cloth (Use Water/Cleaner)										
Vacuum/Hoover Between Bedroom Furniture And The Walls										
Clean And Sanitize Resident's Personal Wheelchair										
Check For Broken Wheelchairs, Frames and Wheels										
Vacuum Under Furniture, Beds, Sofas and Dressers										
Vacuum And Hoover The Carpets, Mats And Rugs										
Vacuum Furnishings, Cushions, Chairs, Sofas And Couches										
Steam Clean Carpets And Rugs										
Dust And Clean Any Picture Frames And Photo Frames										
Ledges, Flat Surfaces And The Tops Of Wardrobes Dusted										
Clean & Check Contents Of Medicine Trolleys & Cupboards										
Clean And Sanitize Mobile Phone, Phone Case And Screen										
Clean & Vacuum The Desk Chair, Legs And Chair Wheels										
Wash And Clean Air Vents										
Dust Ceiling Fan Blades With Duster Or A Microfibre Cloth										
Wash And Clean Windows (Inside And Outside)										
Dust And Clean The Walls From Top To Bottom										
Clean Blinds (Dust The Blinds With A Damp Microfibre Cloth)										
Clean Curtains (Vacuum On A Low Setting Or Wash If Possible)										
Dust And Wash Radiator Covers										
Wash And Clean Ceiling Light Covers										
Clean & Vacuum Central Heating Units (Backs Of Radiators)										
Clean And Disinfect Any Handrails										
Hand Towels Replaced With Fresh Clean Ones										
Sink Wall Mirror Cleaned With Glass Cleaner										
Sinks, Taps And Fixtures Cleaned And Disinfected										
Pour Drain Cleaner Down Sink Drains										
Check For Broken Furniture (Report/Schedule Maintenance)										
Light Bulbs Checked And None Functioning Bulbs Replaced										
Check Hardware, Door Stops And Lock Mechanisms										
Fire Exit Lights And Emergency Lights Checked & Functioning										
Test Carbon Monoxide Alarm And Replace Batteries If Required										
Test Smoke Detector Alarm And Replace Batteries If Required										
Paper Dispensers And Paper Towel Rolls Re-Stocked										
Soap Dispensers, Hand Sanitizers And Hand Gels Are Refilled										
Face Masks, Protective Gloves And Face Shields Re-Stocked										

CARE HOME COMMUNAL AREA CLEANING *Checklist*

Building	Location	Room Number	Area

Start Date & Time	Finnish Date & Time	Name	Signature

	Care Home Cleaning Tasks - Communal Area	M	T	W	T	F	S	S	Cleaned By	Checked By	Date/Tim
1	Clean And Sanitize All The Desks And Tables										
2	Clean And Sanitize All The Counter Tops And Surface Areas										
3	Wipe Down The Walls Wherever There Are Spills And Splashes										
4	Disinfect Touch Points, Light Switches And Other Switches										
5	Clean And Disinfect All Doors, Handles And Doorknobs										
6	Clean And Dust Door Frames, Remember To Dust The Tops										
7	Dust Light Fixtures & Shades With A Duster Or A Microfibre Cloth										
8	Clean And Wipe Mirrors Remove Fingerprints, Smears & Dirt										
9	Clean And Sanitize Over Chair Tables										
10	Clean And Polish Bookshelves, Remember To Dust The Top										
11	Remove, Wash And Clean Any Dirty Cups Or Glasses										
12	Remove, Wash And Clean Any Dirty Plates, Bowels Or Cutlery										
13	Clean And Sanitize Any Chairs, Seats And Benches										
14	Water Jugs (Washed Thoroughly Each Day & Re-Filled)										
15	Water Any Plants And Flowers										
16	Dust Plant Leafs (A Healthy Plant Needs To Be Clear Of Dust)										
17	Empty The Waste Baskets And Recycling Bins										
18	Clean And Disinfectant The Waste Bins And Recycling Bins										
19	Clean And Wipe Down Windowsills										
20	Spray Air Freshener This Keeps The Room Smelling Fresh										
21	Clean And Disinfect Cabinets And Units										
22	Clean And Sanitize Desk Accessories										
23	Replace Dirty Table Linen And Move To Laundry Room										
24	Polish Any Wooden Furniture And Hardwood Surfaces										
25	Clean Skirting Boards/Baseboards And Corners										
26	Clean And Polish Fireplace Mantelpiece And Surrounds										
27	Wipe Down Equipment & Sanitize Tea And Coffee Making Facilities										
28	Clean And Sanitize Telephones, Cords/Leads & All Touch Points										
29	Clean And Sanitize Walking Sticks And Any Other Walking Aids										

Care Home Cleaning Tasks - Communal Area	M	T	W	T	F	S	S	Cleaned By	Checked By	Date/Time
Dust Television, Top Sides And Back, TV Unit And TV Stand										
Clean TV Screen With Soft Damp Cloth (Use Water/Cleaner)										
Vacuum/Hoover Between Furniture And The Walls										
Clean And Sanitize All Wheelchairs										
Check For Broken Wheelchairs, Frames and Wheels										
Vacuum Under Furniture, Units, Tables And Cabinets										
Vacuum And Hoover The Carpets, Mats And Rugs										
Vacuum Furnishings, Cushions, Chairs, Sofas And Couches										
Steam Clean Carpets And Rugs										
Dust And Clean Any Picture Frames And Wall Art										
Clean & Check Contents Of Medicine Trolleys & Cupboards										
Clean & Vacuum The Desk Chair, Legs And Chair Wheels										
Wash And Clean Air Vents										
Dust Ceiling Fan Blades With Duster Or A Microfibre Cloth										
Wash And Clean Windows (Inside And Outside)										
Dust And Clean The Walls From Top To Bottom										
Clean Blinds (Dust The Blinds With A Damp Microfibre Cloth)										
Clean Curtains (Vacuum On A Low Setting Or Wash If Possible)										
Dust And Wash Radiator Covers										
Wash And Clean Ceiling Light Covers										
Clean & Vacuum Central Heating Units (Backs Of Radiators)										
Clean And Disinfect Any Handrails										
Clean And Sanitize Computer, Keyboard And Computer Mice										
Clean And Sanitize iPads, Tablets, Laptops & Mobile Phones										
Floors Mopped Clean With Cleaning Or Disinfecting Solution										
The Floors Are Swept And Free From Debris And Litter										
Clean Sliding Doors and Room Partitions										
Throw Away Outdated Newspapers, Magazines, Papers										
Check For Broken Furniture (Report/Schedule Maintenance)										
Light Bulbs Checked And None Functioning Bulbs Replaced										
Check Hardware, Door Stops And Lock Mechanisms										
Fire Exit Lights And Emergency Lights Checked & Functioning										
Test Carbon Monoxide Alarm And Replace Batteries If Required										
Test Smoke Detector Alarm And Replace Batteries If Required										
Paper Dispensers And Paper Towel Rolls Re-Stocked										
Soap Dispensers, Hand Sanitizers And Hand Gels Are Refilled										
Face Masks, Protective Gloves And Face Shields Re-Stocked										

CARE HOME TOILET & RESTROOM CLEANING *Checklist*

Building	Location	Room Number	Area

Start Date & Time	Finnish Date & Time	Name	Signature

	Care Home Cleaning Tasks - Toilet & Restroom	M	T	W	T	F	S	S	Cleaned By	Checked By	Date/Tim
1	Clean And Sanitize All The Counter Tops And Surface Areas										
2	Wipe Down The Walls Wherever There Are Spills And Splashes										
3	Disinfect Touch Points, Light Switches And Other Switches										
4	Clean And Disinfect All Doors, Handles And Doorknobs										
5	Clean And Dust Door Frames, Remember To Dust The Tops										
6	Dust Light Fixtures With A Duster Or A Microfibre Cloth										
7	Wall Mirrors Cleaned With Glass Cleaner										
8	Clean Any Bathroom Glasses And Cups										
9	Clean And Sanitize Any Chairs And Seats										
10	Empty The Waste Basket And Recycling Bin										
11	Clean And Disinfectant The Waste Bin And Recycling Bin										
12	Clean And Wipe Down Windowsills										
13	Spray Air Freshener This Keeps The Room Smelling Fresh										
14	Air/Odour Control Systems Are Filled And Operating Correctly										
15	Clean Skirting Boards/Baseboards And Corners										
16	Vacuum And Hoover Bath Mats, Shower Mats And Rugs										
17	Replace Bath Mats, Shower Mats And Rugs With Clean Ones										
18	Steam Clean Carpets And Rugs										
19	Hand Towels Replaced With Fresh Clean Ones										
20	Bath Towels Replaced With Fresh Clean Ones										
21	Face Towels Replaced With Fresh Clean Ones										
22	Electric Hand Dryers Cleaned, Disinfected & Operating Correctly										
23	Soap Dispensers, Sanitizers And Hand Gels Are Refilled										
24	Clean & Check Contents Of Medicine Trolleys & Cupboards										
25	Clean And Disinfect Any Handrails										
26	Sinks, Taps And Fixtures Cleaned And Disinfected										
27	Clean And Disinfect Cabinets And Units										
28	Feminine Hygiene Dispensers Re-Stocked										
29	Feminine Hygiene Bins/Containers Emptied And Cleared										

Care Home Cleaning Tasks - Toilet & Restroom	M	T	W	T	F	S	S	Cleaned By	Checked By	Date/Time
Clean & Vacuum Central Heating Units (Backs Of Radiators)										
Wash And Clean Ceiling Light Covers										
Toilet Roll Holders And Toilet Rolls Re-Stocked										
Toilet Roll Holders Cleaned And Disinfected										
Clean Inside The Toilets And Urinals With Disinfectant										
Toilet Seats Cleaned And Disinfected										
Clean Top Of Toilets Tanks, The Bases And Behind Toilets										
Urinal Handles Cleaned And Disinfected										
Urinal Screens Cleaned, Disinfected And Blocks Replaced										
Paper Dispensers And Paper Towel Rolls Re-Stocked										
Paper Dispensers And Paper Towel Roll Cleaned & Disinfected										
The Floors Are Swept And Free From Debris And Litter										
Floors Mopped Clean With Cleaning Or Disinfecting Solution										
Put Up Or Place Wet Floor Signs After Mopping Floors										
Showers And Shower Heads, Cleaned And Disinfected										
Soak Shower Heads										
Clean And Disinfect Glass Shower Doors/Outer Doors										
Clean Soap Scum From Shower Walls										
Clean Blinds (Dust The Blinds With A Damp Microfibre Cloth)										
Clean Curtains (Vacuum On A Low Setting Or Wash If Possible)										
Dust And Wash Radiator Covers										
Clean And Disinfect Commodes Between Each Use										
Clean And Disinfect Shower Chairs Between Each Use										
Bath Hoists Cleaned And Disinfected Between Each Use										
Scrub Tub/Bath, Polish Facets And Taps, Clean & Disinfected										
Toothbrush Holders And Soap Holders Cleaned										
Re-Place Shower Curtains With Clean Fresh Ones										
Wash And Clean Air Vents										
Thoroughly Clean Grout And Tiles										
Disinfect And Clean All The Walls From Top To Bottom										
Wash And Clean Windows (Inside And Outside)										
Unclog The Drains (Sink, Bath And Shower)										
Pour Drain Cleaner Down Sink, Shower & Bath Drains										
Floor Drains And Drain Covers Are Open And Free Of Debris										
Hair Dryers Cleaned And Disinfected And Operating Correctly										
Light Bulbs Checked And None Functioning Bulbs Replaced										
Check Hardware, Door Stops And Lock Mechanisms										

CARE HOME BEDROOM CLEANING *Checklist*

Building	Location	Room Number	Area

Start Date & Time	Finnish Date & Time	Name	Signature

	Care Home Cleaning Tasks - Bedrooms	M	T	W	T	F	S	S	Cleaned By	Checked By	Date/Tim
1	Clean And Sanitize All The Desks And Tables										
2	Clean And Sanitize All The Counter Tops And Surface Areas										
3	Wipe Down The Walls Wherever There Are Spills And Splashes										
4	Disinfect Touch Points, Light Switches And Other Switches										
5	Clean And Disinfect All Doors, Handles And Doorknobs										
6	Clean And Dust Door Frames, Remember To Dust The Tops										
7	Dust Light Fixtures With A Duster Or A Microfibre Cloth										
8	Clean & Wipe Mirrors Remove Fingerprints, Smears & Dirt										
9	Clean And Dust Bedside Cabinets										
10	Clean And Sanitize Over Chair Tables										
11	Clean And Sanitize Over Bed Tables										
12	Clean And Check Bed Frames										
13	Mattresses Hoovered And Cleaned With Disinfectant										
14	Clean And Polish Bookshelves, Remember To Dust The Top										
15	Remove, Wash And Clean Any Dirty Cups Or Glasses										
16	Remove, Wash And Clean Any Dirty Plates, Bowels Or Cutlery										
17	Clean And Sanitize Any Chairs And Seats										
18	Water Jug (Washed Thoroughly Each Day & Re-Filled)										
19	Water Any Plants And Flowers										
20	Dust Plant Leafs (A Healthy Plant Needs To Be Clear Of Dust)										
21	Empty The Waste Basket And Recycling Bin										
22	Clean And Disinfectant The Waste Bin And Recycling Bin										
23	Clean And Wipe Down Windowsills										
24	Spray Air Freshener This Keeps The Room Smelling Fresh										
25	Clean And Disinfect Cabinets And Units										
26	Clean And Sanitize Desk Accessories										
27	Replace Dirty Linen And Move To Laundry Room										
28	Polish Any Wooden Furniture And Hardwood Surfaces										
29	Clean Skirting Boards/Baseboards And Corners										

Care Home Cleaning Tasks - Bedrooms Continued	M	T	W	T	F	S	S	Cleaned By	Checked By	Date/Time
Dust Television, Top Sides And Back, TV Unit And TV Stand										
Clean TV Screen With Soft Damp Cloth (Use Water/Cleaner)										
Vacuum/Hoover Between Bedroom Furniture And The Walls										
Clean And Sanitize Resident's Personal Wheelchair										
Check For Broken Wheelchairs, Frames and Wheels										
Vacuum Under Furniture, Beds, Sofas and Dressers										
Vacuum And Hoover The Carpets, Mats And Rugs										
Vacuum Furnishings, Cushions, Chairs, Sofas And Couches										
Steam Clean Carpets And Rugs										
Dust And Clean Any Picture Frames And Photo Frames										
Ledges, Flat Surfaces And The Tops Of Wardrobes Dusted										
Clean & Check Contents Of Medicine Trolleys & Cupboards										
Clean And Sanitize Mobile Phone, Phone Case And Screen										
Clean & Vacuum The Desk Chair, Legs And Chair Wheels										
Wash And Clean Air Vents										
Dust Ceiling Fan Blades With Duster Or A Microfibre Cloth										
Wash And Clean Windows (Inside And Outside)										
Dust And Clean The Walls From Top To Bottom										
Clean Blinds (Dust The Blinds With A Damp Microfibre Cloth)										
Clean Curtains (Vacuum On A Low Setting Or Wash If Possible)										
Dust And Wash Radiator Covers										
Wash And Clean Ceiling Light Covers										
Clean & Vacuum Central Heating Units (Backs Of Radiators)										
Clean And Disinfect Any Handrails										
Hand Towels Replaced With Fresh Clean Ones										
Sink Wall Mirror Cleaned With Glass Cleaner										
Sinks, Taps And Fixtures Cleaned And Disinfected										
Pour Drain Cleaner Down Sink Drains										
Check For Broken Furniture (Report/Schedule Maintenance)										
Light Bulbs Checked And None Functioning Bulbs Replaced										
Check Hardware, Door Stops And Lock Mechanisms										
Fire Exit Lights And Emergency Lights Checked & Functioning										
Test Carbon Monoxide Alarm And Replace Batteries If Required										
Test Smoke Detector Alarm And Replace Batteries If Required										
Paper Dispensers And Paper Towel Rolls Re-Stocked										
Soap Dispensers, Hand Sanitizers And Hand Gels Are Refilled										
Face Masks, Protective Gloves And Face Shields Re-Stocked										

CARE HOME COMMUNAL AREA CLEANING *Checklist*

Building	Location	Room Number	Area

Start Date & Time	Finnish Date & Time	Name	Signature

	Care Home Cleaning Tasks - Communal Area	M	T	W	T	F	S	S	Cleaned By	Checked By	Date/Tim
1	Clean And Sanitize All The Desks And Tables										
2	Clean And Sanitize All The Counter Tops And Surface Areas										
3	Wipe Down The Walls Wherever There Are Spills And Splashes										
4	Disinfect Touch Points, Light Switches And Other Switches										
5	Clean And Disinfect All Doors, Handles And Doorknobs										
6	Clean And Dust Door Frames, Remember To Dust The Tops										
7	Dust Light Fixtures & Shades With A Duster Or A Microfibre Cloth										
8	Clean And Wipe Mirrors Remove Fingerprints, Smears & Dirt										
9	Clean And Sanitize Over Chair Tables										
10	Clean And Polish Bookshelves, Remember To Dust The Top										
11	Remove, Wash And Clean Any Dirty Cups Or Glasses										
12	Remove, Wash And Clean Any Dirty Plates, Bowels Or Cutlery										
13	Clean And Sanitize Any Chairs, Seats And Benches										
14	Water Jugs (Washed Thoroughly Each Day & Re-Filled)										
15	Water Any Plants And Flowers										
16	Dust Plant Leafs (A Healthy Plant Needs To Be Clear Of Dust)										
17	Empty The Waste Baskets And Recycling Bins										
18	Clean And Disinfectant The Waste Bins And Recycling Bins										
19	Clean And Wipe Down Windowsills										
20	Spray Air Freshener This Keeps The Room Smelling Fresh										
21	Clean And Disinfect Cabinets And Units										
22	Clean And Sanitize Desk Accessories										
23	Replace Dirty Table Linen And Move To Laundry Room										
24	Polish Any Wooden Furniture And Hardwood Surfaces										
25	Clean Skirting Boards/Baseboards And Corners										
26	Clean And Polish Fireplace Mantelpiece And Surrounds										
27	Wipe Down Equipment & Sanitize Tea And Coffee Making Facilities										
28	Clean And Sanitize Telephones, Cords/Leads & All Touch Points										
29	Clean And Sanitize Walking Sticks And Any Other Walking Aids										

Care Home Cleaning Tasks - Communal Area	M	T	W	T	F	S	S	Cleaned By	Checked By	Date/Time
Dust Television, Top Sides And Back, TV Unit And TV Stand										
Clean TV Screen With Soft Damp Cloth (Use Water/Cleaner)										
Vacuum/Hoover Between Furniture And The Walls										
Clean And Sanitize All Wheelchairs										
Check For Broken Wheelchairs, Frames and Wheels										
Vacuum Under Furniture, Units, Tables And Cabinets										
Vacuum And Hoover The Carpets, Mats And Rugs										
Vacuum Furnishings, Cushions, Chairs, Sofas And Couches										
Steam Clean Carpets And Rugs										
Dust And Clean Any Picture Frames And Wall Art										
Clean & Check Contents Of Medicine Trolleys & Cupboards										
Clean & Vacuum The Desk Chair, Legs And Chair Wheels										
Wash And Clean Air Vents										
Dust Ceiling Fan Blades With Duster Or A Microfibre Cloth										
Wash And Clean Windows (Inside And Outside)										
Dust And Clean The Walls From Top To Bottom										
Clean Blinds (Dust The Blinds With A Damp Microfibre Cloth)										
Clean Curtains (Vacuum On A Low Setting Or Wash If Possible)										
Dust And Wash Radiator Covers										
Wash And Clean Ceiling Light Covers										
Clean & Vacuum Central Heating Units (Backs Of Radiators)										
Clean And Disinfect Any Handrails										
Clean And Sanitize Computer, Keyboard And Computer Mice										
Clean And Sanitize iPads, Tablets, Laptops & Mobile Phones										
Floors Mopped Clean With Cleaning Or Disinfecting Solution										
The Floors Are Swept And Free From Debris And Litter										
Clean Sliding Doors and Room Partitions										
Throw Away Outdated Newspapers, Magazines, Papers										
Check For Broken Furniture (Report/Schedule Maintenance)										
Light Bulbs Checked And None Functioning Bulbs Replaced										
Check Hardware, Door Stops And Lock Mechanisms										
Fire Exit Lights And Emergency Lights Checked & Functioning										
Test Carbon Monoxide Alarm And Replace Batteries If Required										
Test Smoke Detector Alarm And Replace Batteries If Required										
Paper Dispensers And Paper Towel Rolls Re-Stocked										
Soap Dispensers, Hand Sanitizers And Hand Gels Are Refilled										
Face Masks, Protective Gloves And Face Shields Re-Stocked										

CARE HOME TOILET & RESTROOM CLEANING *Checklist*

Building	Location	Room Number	Area

Start Date & Time	Finnish Date & Time	Name	Signature

	Care Home Cleaning Tasks - Toilet & Restroom	M	T	W	T	F	S	S	Cleaned By	Checked By	Date/Time
1	Clean And Sanitize All The Counter Tops And Surface Areas										
2	Wipe Down The Walls Wherever There Are Spills And Splashes										
3	Disinfect Touch Points, Light Switches And Other Switches										
4	Clean And Disinfect All Doors, Handles And Doorknobs										
5	Clean And Dust Door Frames, Remember To Dust The Tops										
6	Dust Light Fixtures With A Duster Or A Microfibre Cloth										
7	Wall Mirrors Cleaned With Glass Cleaner										
8	Clean Any Bathroom Glasses And Cups										
9	Clean And Sanitize Any Chairs And Seats										
10	Empty The Waste Basket And Recycling Bin										
11	Clean And Disinfectant The Waste Bin And Recycling Bin										
12	Clean And Wipe Down Windowsills										
13	Spray Air Freshener This Keeps The Room Smelling Fresh										
14	Air/Odour Control Systems Are Filled And Operating Correctly										
15	Clean Skirting Boards/Baseboards And Corners										
16	Vacuum And Hoover Bath Mats, Shower Mats And Rugs										
17	Replace Bath Mats, Shower Mats And Rugs With Clean Ones										
18	Steam Clean Carpets And Rugs										
19	Hand Towels Replaced With Fresh Clean Ones										
20	Bath Towels Replaced With Fresh Clean Ones										
21	Face Towels Replaced With Fresh Clean Ones										
22	Electric Hand Dryers Cleaned, Disinfected & Operating Correctly										
23	Soap Dispensers, Sanitizers And Hand Gels Are Refilled										
24	Clean & Check Contents Of Medicine Trolleys & Cupboards										
25	Clean And Disinfect Any Handrails										
26	Sinks, Taps And Fixtures Cleaned And Disinfected										
27	Clean And Disinfect Cabinets And Units										
28	Feminine Hygiene Dispensers Re-Stocked										
29	Feminine Hygiene Bins/Containers Emptied And Cleared										

Care Home Cleaning Tasks - Toilet & Restroom	M	T	W	T	F	S	S	Cleaned By	Checked By	Date/Time
Clean & Vacuum Central Heating Units (Backs Of Radiators)										
Wash And Clean Ceiling Light Covers										
Toilet Roll Holders And Toilet Rolls Re-Stocked										
Toilet Roll Holders Cleaned And Disinfected										
Clean Inside The Toilets And Urinals With Disinfectant										
Toilet Seats Cleaned And Disinfected										
Clean Top Of Toilets Tanks, The Bases And Behind Toilets										
Urinal Handles Cleaned And Disinfected										
Urinal Screens Cleaned, Disinfected And Blocks Replaced										
Paper Dispensers And Paper Towel Rolls Re-Stocked										
Paper Dispensers And Paper Towel Roll Cleaned & Disinfected										
The Floors Are Swept And Free From Debris And Litter										
Floors Mopped Clean With Cleaning Or Disinfecting Solution										
Put Up Or Place Wet Floor Signs After Mopping Floors										
Showers And Shower Heads, Cleaned And Disinfected										
Soak Shower Heads										
Clean And Disinfect Glass Shower Doors/Outer Doors										
Clean Soap Scum From Shower Walls										
Clean Blinds (Dust The Blinds With A Damp Microfibre Cloth)										
Clean Curtains (Vacuum On A Low Setting Or Wash If Possible)										
Dust And Wash Radiator Covers										
Clean And Disinfect Commodes Between Each Use										
Clean And Disinfect Shower Chairs Between Each Use										
Bath Hoists Cleaned And Disinfected Between Each Use										
Scrub Tub/Bath, Polish Facets And Taps, Clean & Disinfected										
Toothbrush Holders And Soap Holders Cleaned										
Re-Place Shower Curtains With Clean Fresh Ones										
Wash And Clean Air Vents										
Thoroughly Clean Grout And Tiles										
Disinfect And Clean All The Walls From Top To Bottom										
Wash And Clean Windows (Inside And Outside)										
Unclog The Drains (Sink, Bath And Shower)										
Pour Drain Cleaner Down Sink, Shower & Bath Drains										
Floor Drains And Drain Covers Are Open And Free Of Debris										
Hair Dryers Cleaned And Disinfected And Operating Correctly										
Light Bulbs Checked And None Functioning Bulbs Replaced										
Check Hardware, Door Stops And Lock Mechanisms										

CARE HOME BEDROOM CLEANING *Checklist*

Building	Location	Room Number	Area

Start Date & Time	Finnish Date & Time	Name	Signature

	Care Home Cleaning Tasks - Bedrooms	M	T	W	T	F	S	S	Cleaned By	Checked By	Date/Tin
1	Clean And Sanitize All The Desks And Tables										
2	Clean And Sanitize All The Counter Tops And Surface Areas										
3	Wipe Down The Walls Wherever There Are Spills And Splashes										
4	Disinfect Touch Points, Light Switches And Other Switches										
5	Clean And Disinfect All Doors, Handles And Doorknobs										
6	Clean And Dust Door Frames, Remember To Dust The Tops										
7	Dust Light Fixtures With A Duster Or A Microfibre Cloth										
8	Clean & Wipe Mirrors Remove Fingerprints, Smears & Dirt										
9	Clean And Dust Bedside Cabinets										
10	Clean And Sanitize Over Chair Tables										
11	Clean And Sanitize Over Bed Tables										
12	Clean And Check Bed Frames										
13	Mattresses Hoovered And Cleaned With Disinfectant										
14	Clean And Polish Bookshelves, Remember To Dust The Top										
15	Remove, Wash And Clean Any Dirty Cups Or Glasses										
16	Remove, Wash And Clean Any Dirty Plates, Bowels Or Cutlery										
17	Clean And Sanitize Any Chairs And Seats										
18	Water Jug (Washed Thoroughly Each Day & Re-Filled)										
19	Water Any Plants And Flowers										
20	Dust Plant Leafs (A Healthy Plant Needs To Be Clear Of Dust)										
21	Empty The Waste Basket And Recycling Bin										
22	Clean And Disinfectant The Waste Bin And Recycling Bin										
23	Clean And Wipe Down Windowsills										
24	Spray Air Freshener This Keeps The Room Smelling Fresh										
25	Clean And Disinfect Cabinets And Units										
26	Clean And Sanitize Desk Accessories										
27	Replace Dirty Linen And Move To Laundry Room										
28	Polish Any Wooden Furniture And Hardwood Surfaces										
29	Clean Skirting Boards/Baseboards And Corners										

Care Home Cleaning Tasks - Bedrooms Continued	M	T	W	T	F	S	S	Cleaned By	Checked By	Date/Time
Dust Television, Top Sides And Back, TV Unit And TV Stand										
Clean TV Screen With Soft Damp Cloth (Use Water/Cleaner)										
Vacuum/Hoover Between Bedroom Furniture And The Walls										
Clean And Sanitize Resident's Personal Wheelchair										
Check For Broken Wheelchairs, Frames and Wheels										
Vacuum Under Furniture, Beds, Sofas and Dressers										
Vacuum And Hoover The Carpets, Mats And Rugs										
Vacuum Furnishings, Cushions, Chairs, Sofas And Couches										
Steam Clean Carpets And Rugs										
Dust And Clean Any Picture Frames And Photo Frames										
Ledges, Flat Surfaces And The Tops Of Wardrobes Dusted										
Clean & Check Contents Of Medicine Trolleys & Cupboards										
Clean And Sanitize Mobile Phone, Phone Case And Screen										
Clean & Vacuum The Desk Chair, Legs And Chair Wheels										
Wash And Clean Air Vents										
Dust Ceiling Fan Blades With Duster Or A Microfibre Cloth										
Wash And Clean Windows (Inside And Outside)										
Dust And Clean The Walls From Top To Bottom										
Clean Blinds (Dust The Blinds With A Damp Microfibre Cloth)										
Clean Curtains (Vacuum On A Low Setting Or Wash If Possible)										
Dust And Wash Radiator Covers										
Wash And Clean Ceiling Light Covers										
Clean & Vacuum Central Heating Units (Backs Of Radiators)										
Clean And Disinfect Any Handrails										
Hand Towels Replaced With Fresh Clean Ones										
Sink Wall Mirror Cleaned With Glass Cleaner										
Sinks, Taps And Fixtures Cleaned And Disinfected										
Pour Drain Cleaner Down Sink Drains										
Check For Broken Furniture (Report/Schedule Maintenance)										
Light Bulbs Checked And None Functioning Bulbs Replaced										
Check Hardware, Door Stops And Lock Mechanisms										
Fire Exit Lights And Emergency Lights Checked & Functioning										
Test Carbon Monoxide Alarm And Replace Batteries If Required										
Test Smoke Detector Alarm And Replace Batteries If Required										
Paper Dispensers And Paper Towel Rolls Re-Stocked										
Soap Dispensers, Hand Sanitizers And Hand Gels Are Refilled										
Face Masks, Protective Gloves And Face Shields Re-Stocked										

CARE HOME COMMUNAL AREA CLEANING *Checklist*

Building	Location	Room Number	Area

Start Date & Time	Finnish Date & Time	Name	Signature

	Care Home Cleaning Tasks - Communal Area	M	T	W	T	F	S	S	Cleaned By	Checked By	Date/Tim
1	Clean And Sanitize All The Desks And Tables										
2	Clean And Sanitize All The Counter Tops And Surface Areas										
3	Wipe Down The Walls Wherever There Are Spills And Splashes										
4	Disinfect Touch Points, Light Switches And Other Switches										
5	Clean And Disinfect All Doors, Handles And Doorknobs										
6	Clean And Dust Door Frames, Remember To Dust The Tops										
7	Dust Light Fixtures & Shades With A Duster Or A Microfibre Cloth										
8	Clean And Wipe Mirrors Remove Fingerprints, Smears & Dirt										
9	Clean And Sanitize Over Chair Tables										
10	Clean And Polish Bookshelves, Remember To Dust The Top										
11	Remove, Wash And Clean Any Dirty Cups Or Glasses										
12	Remove, Wash And Clean Any Dirty Plates, Bowels Or Cutlery										
13	Clean And Sanitize Any Chairs, Seats And Benches										
14	Water Jugs (Washed Thoroughly Each Day & Re-Filled)										
15	Water Any Plants And Flowers										
16	Dust Plant Leafs (A Healthy Plant Needs To Be Clear Of Dust)										
17	Empty The Waste Baskets And Recycling Bins										
18	Clean And Disinfectant The Waste Bins And Recycling Bins										
19	Clean And Wipe Down Windowsills										
20	Spray Air Freshener This Keeps The Room Smelling Fresh										
21	Clean And Disinfect Cabinets And Units										
22	Clean And Sanitize Desk Accessories										
23	Replace Dirty Table Linen And Move To Laundry Room										
24	Polish Any Wooden Furniture And Hardwood Surfaces										
25	Clean Skirting Boards/Baseboards And Corners										
26	Clean And Polish Fireplace Mantelpiece And Surrounds										
27	Wipe Down Equipment & Sanitize Tea And Coffee Making Facilities										
28	Clean And Sanitize Telephones, Cords/Leads & All Touch Points										
29	Clean And Sanitize Walking Sticks And Any Other Walking Aids										

Care Home Cleaning Tasks - Communal Area	M	T	W	T	F	S	S	Cleaned By	Checked By	Date/Time
Dust Television, Top Sides And Back, TV Unit And TV Stand										
Clean TV Screen With Soft Damp Cloth (Use Water/Cleaner)										
Vacuum/Hoover Between Furniture And The Walls										
Clean And Sanitize All Wheelchairs										
Check For Broken Wheelchairs, Frames and Wheels										
Vacuum Under Furniture, Units, Tables And Cabinets										
Vacuum And Hoover The Carpets, Mats And Rugs										
Vacuum Furnishings, Cushions, Chairs, Sofas And Couches										
Steam Clean Carpets And Rugs										
Dust And Clean Any Picture Frames And Wall Art										
Clean & Check Contents Of Medicine Trolleys & Cupboards										
Clean & Vacuum The Desk Chair, Legs And Chair Wheels										
Wash And Clean Air Vents										
Dust Ceiling Fan Blades With Duster Or A Microfibre Cloth										
Wash And Clean Windows (Inside And Outside)										
Dust And Clean The Walls From Top To Bottom										
Clean Blinds (Dust The Blinds With A Damp Microfibre Cloth)										
Clean Curtains (Vacuum On A Low Setting Or Wash If Possible)										
Dust And Wash Radiator Covers										
Wash And Clean Ceiling Light Covers										
Clean & Vacuum Central Heating Units (Backs Of Radiators)										
Clean And Disinfect Any Handrails										
Clean And Sanitize Computer, Keyboard And Computer Mice										
Clean And Sanitize iPads, Tablets, Laptops & Mobile Phones										
Floors Mopped Clean With Cleaning Or Disinfecting Solution										
The Floors Are Swept And Free From Debris And Litter										
Clean Sliding Doors and Room Partitions										
Throw Away Outdated Newspapers, Magazines, Papers										
Check For Broken Furniture (Report/Schedule Maintenance)										
Light Bulbs Checked And None Functioning Bulbs Replaced										
Check Hardware, Door Stops And Lock Mechanisms										
Fire Exit Lights And Emergency Lights Checked & Functioning										
Test Carbon Monoxide Alarm And Replace Batteries If Required										
Test Smoke Detector Alarm And Replace Batteries If Required										
Paper Dispensers And Paper Towel Rolls Re-Stocked										
Soap Dispensers, Hand Sanitizers And Hand Gels Are Refilled										
Face Masks, Protective Gloves And Face Shields Re-Stocked										

CARE HOME TOILET & RESTROOM CLEANING *Checklist*

Building	Location	Room Number	Area

Start Date & Time	Finnish Date & Time	Name	Signature

	Care Home Cleaning Tasks - Toilet & Restroom	M	T	W	T	F	S	S	Cleaned By	Checked By	Date/Time
1	Clean And Sanitize All The Counter Tops And Surface Areas										
2	Wipe Down The Walls Wherever There Are Spills And Splashes										
3	Disinfect Touch Points, Light Switches And Other Switches										
4	Clean And Disinfect All Doors, Handles And Doorknobs										
5	Clean And Dust Door Frames, Remember To Dust The Tops										
6	Dust Light Fixtures With A Duster Or A Microfibre Cloth										
7	Wall Mirrors Cleaned With Glass Cleaner										
8	Clean Any Bathroom Glasses And Cups										
9	Clean And Sanitize Any Chairs And Seats										
10	Empty The Waste Basket And Recycling Bin										
11	Clean And Disinfectant The Waste Bin And Recycling Bin										
12	Clean And Wipe Down Windowsills										
13	Spray Air Freshener This Keeps The Room Smelling Fresh										
14	Air/Odour Control Systems Are Filled And Operating Correctly										
15	Clean Skirting Boards/Baseboards And Corners										
16	Vacuum And Hoover Bath Mats, Shower Mats And Rugs										
17	Replace Bath Mats, Shower Mats And Rugs With Clean Ones										
18	Steam Clean Carpets And Rugs										
19	Hand Towels Replaced With Fresh Clean Ones										
20	Bath Towels Replaced With Fresh Clean Ones										
21	Face Towels Replaced With Fresh Clean Ones										
22	Electric Hand Dryers Cleaned, Disinfected & Operating Correctly										
23	Soap Dispensers, Sanitizers And Hand Gels Are Refilled										
24	Clean & Check Contents Of Medicine Trolleys & Cupboards										
25	Clean And Disinfect Any Handrails										
26	Sinks, Taps And Fixtures Cleaned And Disinfected										
27	Clean And Disinfect Cabinets And Units										
28	Feminine Hygiene Dispensers Re-Stocked										
29	Feminine Hygiene Bins/Containers Emptied And Cleared										

Care Home Cleaning Tasks - Toilet & Restroom	M	T	W	T	F	S	S	Cleaned By	Checked By	Date/Time
Clean & Vacuum Central Heating Units (Backs Of Radiators)										
Wash And Clean Ceiling Light Covers										
Toilet Roll Holders And Toilet Rolls Re-Stocked										
Toilet Roll Holders Cleaned And Disinfected										
Clean Inside The Toilets And Urinals With Disinfectant										
Toilet Seats Cleaned And Disinfected										
Clean Top Of Toilets Tanks, The Bases And Behind Toilets										
Urinal Handles Cleaned And Disinfected										
Urinal Screens Cleaned, Disinfected And Blocks Replaced										
Paper Dispensers And Paper Towel Rolls Re-Stocked										
Paper Dispensers And Paper Towel Roll Cleaned & Disinfected										
The Floors Are Swept And Free From Debris And Litter										
Floors Mopped Clean With Cleaning Or Disinfecting Solution										
Put Up Or Place Wet Floor Signs After Mopping Floors										
Showers And Shower Heads, Cleaned And Disinfected										
Soak Shower Heads										
Clean And Disinfect Glass Shower Doors/Outer Doors										
Clean Soap Scum From Shower Walls										
Clean Blinds (Dust The Blinds With A Damp Microfibre Cloth)										
Clean Curtains (Vacuum On A Low Setting Or Wash If Possible)										
Dust And Wash Radiator Covers										
Clean And Disinfect Commodes Between Each Use										
Clean And Disinfect Shower Chairs Between Each Use										
Bath Hoists Cleaned And Disinfected Between Each Use										
Scrub Tub/Bath, Polish Facets And Taps, Clean & Disinfected										
Toothbrush Holders And Soap Holders Cleaned										
Re-Place Shower Curtains With Clean Fresh Ones										
Wash And Clean Air Vents										
Thoroughly Clean Grout And Tiles										
Disinfect And Clean All The Walls From Top To Bottom										
Wash And Clean Windows (Inside And Outside)										
Unclog The Drains (Sink, Bath And Shower)										
Pour Drain Cleaner Down Sink, Shower & Bath Drains										
Floor Drains And Drain Covers Are Open And Free Of Debris										
Hair Dryers Cleaned And Disinfected And Operating Correctly										
Light Bulbs Checked And None Functioning Bulbs Replaced										
Check Hardware, Door Stops And Lock Mechanisms										

CARE HOME BEDROOM CLEANING *Checklist*

Building	Location	Room Number	Area

Start Date & Time	Finnish Date & Time	Name	Signature

	Care Home Cleaning Tasks - Bedrooms	M	T	W	T	F	S	S	Cleaned By	Checked By	Date/Tim
1	Clean And Sanitize All The Desks And Tables										
2	Clean And Sanitize All The Counter Tops And Surface Areas										
3	Wipe Down The Walls Wherever There Are Spills And Splashes										
4	Disinfect Touch Points, Light Switches And Other Switches										
5	Clean And Disinfect All Doors, Handles And Doorknobs										
6	Clean And Dust Door Frames, Remember To Dust The Tops										
7	Dust Light Fixtures With A Duster Or A Microfibre Cloth										
8	Clean & Wipe Mirrors Remove Fingerprints, Smears & Dirt										
9	Clean And Dust Bedside Cabinets										
10	Clean And Sanitize Over Chair Tables										
11	Clean And Sanitize Over Bed Tables										
12	Clean And Check Bed Frames										
13	Mattresses Hoovered And Cleaned With Disinfectant										
14	Clean And Polish Bookshelves, Remember To Dust The Top										
15	Remove, Wash And Clean Any Dirty Cups Or Glasses										
16	Remove, Wash And Clean Any Dirty Plates, Bowels Or Cutlery										
17	Clean And Sanitize Any Chairs And Seats										
18	Water Jug (Washed Thoroughly Each Day & Re-Filled)										
19	Water Any Plants And Flowers										
20	Dust Plant Leafs (A Healthy Plant Needs To Be Clear Of Dust)										
21	Empty The Waste Basket And Recycling Bin										
22	Clean And Disinfectant The Waste Bin And Recycling Bin										
23	Clean And Wipe Down Windowsills										
24	Spray Air Freshener This Keeps The Room Smelling Fresh										
25	Clean And Disinfect Cabinets And Units										
26	Clean And Sanitize Desk Accessories										
27	Replace Dirty Linen And Move To Laundry Room										
28	Polish Any Wooden Furniture And Hardwood Surfaces										
29	Clean Skirting Boards/Baseboards And Corners										

Care Home Cleaning Tasks - Bedrooms Continued	M	T	W	T	F	S	S	Cleaned By	Checked By	Date/Time
Dust Television, Top Sides And Back, TV Unit And TV Stand										
Clean TV Screen With Soft Damp Cloth (Use Water/Cleaner)										
Vacuum/Hoover Between Bedroom Furniture And The Walls										
Clean And Sanitize Resident's Personal Wheelchair										
Check For Broken Wheelchairs, Frames and Wheels										
Vacuum Under Furniture, Beds, Sofas and Dressers										
Vacuum And Hoover The Carpets, Mats And Rugs										
Vacuum Furnishings, Cushions, Chairs, Sofas And Couches										
Steam Clean Carpets And Rugs										
Dust And Clean Any Picture Frames And Photo Frames										
Ledges, Flat Surfaces And The Tops Of Wardrobes Dusted										
Clean & Check Contents Of Medicine Trolleys & Cupboards										
Clean And Sanitize Mobile Phone, Phone Case And Screen										
Clean & Vacuum The Desk Chair, Legs And Chair Wheels										
Wash And Clean Air Vents										
Dust Ceiling Fan Blades With Duster Or A Microfibre Cloth										
Wash And Clean Windows (Inside And Outside)										
Dust And Clean The Walls From Top To Bottom										
Clean Blinds (Dust The Blinds With A Damp Microfibre Cloth)										
Clean Curtains (Vacuum On A Low Setting Or Wash If Possible)										
Dust And Wash Radiator Covers										
Wash And Clean Ceiling Light Covers										
Clean & Vacuum Central Heating Units (Backs Of Radiators)										
Clean And Disinfect Any Handrails										
Hand Towels Replaced With Fresh Clean Ones										
Sink Wall Mirror Cleaned With Glass Cleaner										
Sinks, Taps And Fixtures Cleaned And Disinfected										
Pour Drain Cleaner Down Sink Drains										
Check For Broken Furniture (Report/Schedule Maintenance)										
Light Bulbs Checked And None Functioning Bulbs Replaced										
Check Hardware, Door Stops And Lock Mechanisms										
Fire Exit Lights And Emergency Lights Checked & Functioning										
Test Carbon Monoxide Alarm And Replace Batteries If Required										
Test Smoke Detector Alarm And Replace Batteries If Required										
Paper Dispensers And Paper Towel Rolls Re-Stocked										
Soap Dispensers, Hand Sanitizers And Hand Gels Are Refilled										
Face Masks, Protective Gloves And Face Shields Re-Stocked										

CARE HOME COMMUNAL AREA CLEANING *Checklist*

Building	Location	Room Number	Area

Start Date & Time	Finnish Date & Time	Name	Signature

	Care Home Cleaning Tasks - Communal Area	M	T	W	T	F	S	S	Cleaned By	Checked By	Date/Tim
1	Clean And Sanitize All The Desks And Tables										
2	Clean And Sanitize All The Counter Tops And Surface Areas										
3	Wipe Down The Walls Wherever There Are Spills And Splashes										
4	Disinfect Touch Points, Light Switches And Other Switches										
5	Clean And Disinfect All Doors, Handles And Doorknobs										
6	Clean And Dust Door Frames, Remember To Dust The Tops										
7	Dust Light Fixtures & Shades With A Duster Or A Microfibre Cloth										
8	Clean And Wipe Mirrors Remove Fingerprints, Smears & Dirt										
9	Clean And Sanitize Over Chair Tables										
10	Clean And Polish Bookshelves, Remember To Dust The Top										
11	Remove, Wash And Clean Any Dirty Cups Or Glasses										
12	Remove, Wash And Clean Any Dirty Plates, Bowels Or Cutlery										
13	Clean And Sanitize Any Chairs, Seats And Benches										
14	Water Jugs (Washed Thoroughly Each Day & Re-Filled)										
15	Water Any Plants And Flowers										
16	Dust Plant Leafs (A Healthy Plant Needs To Be Clear Of Dust)										
17	Empty The Waste Baskets And Recycling Bins										
18	Clean And Disinfectant The Waste Bins And Recycling Bins										
19	Clean And Wipe Down Windowsills										
20	Spray Air Freshener This Keeps The Room Smelling Fresh										
21	Clean And Disinfect Cabinets And Units										
22	Clean And Sanitize Desk Accessories										
23	Replace Dirty Table Linen And Move To Laundry Room										
24	Polish Any Wooden Furniture And Hardwood Surfaces										
25	Clean Skirting Boards/Baseboards And Corners										
26	Clean And Polish Fireplace Mantelpiece And Surrounds										
27	Wipe Down Equipment & Sanitize Tea And Coffee Making Facilities										
28	Clean And Sanitize Telephones, Cords/Leads & All Touch Points										
29	Clean And Sanitize Walking Sticks And Any Other Walking Aids										

Care Home Cleaning Tasks - Communal Area	M	T	W	T	F	S	S	Cleaned By	Checked By	Date/Time
Dust Television, Top Sides And Back, TV Unit And TV Stand										
Clean TV Screen With Soft Damp Cloth (Use Water/Cleaner)										
Vacuum/Hoover Between Furniture And The Walls										
Clean And Sanitize All Wheelchairs										
Check For Broken Wheelchairs, Frames and Wheels										
Vacuum Under Furniture, Units, Tables And Cabinets										
Vacuum And Hoover The Carpets, Mats And Rugs										
Vacuum Furnishings, Cushions, Chairs, Sofas And Couches										
Steam Clean Carpets And Rugs										
Dust And Clean Any Picture Frames And Wall Art										
Clean & Check Contents Of Medicine Trolleys & Cupboards										
Clean & Vacuum The Desk Chair, Legs And Chair Wheels										
Wash And Clean Air Vents										
Dust Ceiling Fan Blades With Duster Or A Microfibre Cloth										
Wash And Clean Windows (Inside And Outside)										
Dust And Clean The Walls From Top To Bottom										
Clean Blinds (Dust The Blinds With A Damp Microfibre Cloth)										
Clean Curtains (Vacuum On A Low Setting Or Wash If Possible)										
Dust And Wash Radiator Covers										
Wash And Clean Ceiling Light Covers										
Clean & Vacuum Central Heating Units (Backs Of Radiators)										
Clean And Disinfect Any Handrails										
Clean And Sanitize Computer, Keyboard And Computer Mice										
Clean And Sanitize iPads, Tablets, Laptops & Mobile Phones										
Floors Mopped Clean With Cleaning Or Disinfecting Solution										
The Floors Are Swept And Free From Debris And Litter										
Clean Sliding Doors and Room Partitions										
Throw Away Outdated Newspapers, Magazines, Papers										
Check For Broken Furniture (Report/Schedule Maintenance)										
Light Bulbs Checked And None Functioning Bulbs Replaced										
Check Hardware, Door Stops And Lock Mechanisms										
Fire Exit Lights And Emergency Lights Checked & Functioning										
Test Carbon Monoxide Alarm And Replace Batteries If Required										
Test Smoke Detector Alarm And Replace Batteries If Required										
Paper Dispensers And Paper Towel Rolls Re-Stocked										
Soap Dispensers, Hand Sanitizers And Hand Gels Are Refilled										
Face Masks, Protective Gloves And Face Shields Re-Stocked										

CARE HOME TOILET & RESTROOM CLEANING *Checklis*

Building	Location	Room Number	Area

Start Date & Time	Finnish Date & Time	Name	Signature

	Care Home Cleaning Tasks - Toilet & Restroom	M	T	W	T	F	S	S	Cleaned By	Checked By	Date/Tim
1	Clean And Sanitize All The Counter Tops And Surface Areas										
2	Wipe Down The Walls Wherever There Are Spills And Splashes										
3	Disinfect Touch Points, Light Switches And Other Switches										
4	Clean And Disinfect All Doors, Handles And Doorknobs										
5	Clean And Dust Door Frames, Remember To Dust The Tops										
6	Dust Light Fixtures With A Duster Or A Microfibre Cloth										
7	Wall Mirrors Cleaned With Glass Cleaner										
8	Clean Any Bathroom Glasses And Cups										
9	Clean And Sanitize Any Chairs And Seats										
10	Empty The Waste Basket And Recycling Bin										
11	Clean And Disinfectant The Waste Bin And Recycling Bin										
12	Clean And Wipe Down Windowsills										
13	Spray Air Freshener This Keeps The Room Smelling Fresh										
14	Air/Odour Control Systems Are Filled And Operating Correctly										
15	Clean Skirting Boards/Baseboards And Corners										
16	Vacuum And Hoover Bath Mats, Shower Mats And Rugs										
17	Replace Bath Mats, Shower Mats And Rugs With Clean Ones										
18	Steam Clean Carpets And Rugs										
19	Hand Towels Replaced With Fresh Clean Ones										
20	Bath Towels Replaced With Fresh Clean Ones										
21	Face Towels Replaced With Fresh Clean Ones										
22	Electric Hand Dryers Cleaned, Disinfected & Operating Correctly										
23	Soap Dispensers, Sanitizers And Hand Gels Are Refilled										
24	Clean & Check Contents Of Medicine Trolleys & Cupboards										
25	Clean And Disinfect Any Handrails										
26	Sinks, Taps And Fixtures Cleaned And Disinfected										
27	Clean And Disinfect Cabinets And Units										
28	Feminine Hygiene Dispensers Re-Stocked										
29	Feminine Hygiene Bins/Containers Emptied And Cleared										

Care Home Cleaning Tasks - Toilet & Restroom	M	T	W	T	F	S	S	Cleaned By	Checked By	Date/Time
Clean & Vacuum Central Heating Units (Backs Of Radiators)										
Wash And Clean Ceiling Light Covers										
Toilet Roll Holders And Toilet Rolls Re-Stocked										
Toilet Roll Holders Cleaned And Disinfected										
Clean Inside The Toilets And Urinals With Disinfectant										
Toilet Seats Cleaned And Disinfected										
Clean Top Of Toilets Tanks, The Bases And Behind Toilets										
Urinal Handles Cleaned And Disinfected										
Urinal Screens Cleaned, Disinfected And Blocks Replaced										
Paper Dispensers And Paper Towel Rolls Re-Stocked										
Paper Dispensers And Paper Towel Roll Cleaned & Disinfected										
The Floors Are Swept And Free From Debris And Litter										
Floors Mopped Clean With Cleaning Or Disinfecting Solution										
Put Up Or Place Wet Floor Signs After Mopping Floors										
Showers And Shower Heads, Cleaned And Disinfected										
Soak Shower Heads										
Clean And Disinfect Glass Shower Doors/Outer Doors										
Clean Soap Scum From Shower Walls										
Clean Blinds (Dust The Blinds With A Damp Microfibre Cloth)										
Clean Curtains (Vacuum On A Low Setting Or Wash If Possible)										
Dust And Wash Radiator Covers										
Clean And Disinfect Commodes Between Each Use										
Clean And Disinfect Shower Chairs Between Each Use										
Bath Hoists Cleaned And Disinfected Between Each Use										
Scrub Tub/Bath, Polish Facets And Taps, Clean & Disinfected										
Toothbrush Holders And Soap Holders Cleaned										
Re-Place Shower Curtains With Clean Fresh Ones										
Wash And Clean Air Vents										
Thoroughly Clean Grout And Tiles										
Disinfect And Clean All The Walls From Top To Bottom										
Wash And Clean Windows (Inside And Outside)										
Unclog The Drains (Sink, Bath And Shower)										
Pour Drain Cleaner Down Sink, Shower & Bath Drains										
Floor Drains And Drain Covers Are Open And Free Of Debris										
Hair Dryers Cleaned And Disinfected And Operating Correctly										
Light Bulbs Checked And None Functioning Bulbs Replaced										
Check Hardware, Door Stops And Lock Mechanisms										

CARE HOME BEDROOM CLEANING *Checklist*

Building	Location	Room Number	Area

Start Date & Time	Finnish Date & Time	Name	Signature

	Care Home Cleaning Tasks - Bedrooms	M	T	W	T	F	S	S	Cleaned By	Checked By	Date/Tim
1	Clean And Sanitize All The Desks And Tables										
2	Clean And Sanitize All The Counter Tops And Surface Areas										
3	Wipe Down The Walls Wherever There Are Spills And Splashes										
4	Disinfect Touch Points, Light Switches And Other Switches										
5	Clean And Disinfect All Doors, Handles And Doorknobs										
6	Clean And Dust Door Frames, Remember To Dust The Tops										
7	Dust Light Fixtures With A Duster Or A Microfibre Cloth										
8	Clean & Wipe Mirrors Remove Fingerprints, Smears & Dirt										
9	Clean And Dust Bedside Cabinets										
10	Clean And Sanitize Over Chair Tables										
11	Clean And Sanitize Over Bed Tables										
12	Clean And Check Bed Frames										
13	Mattresses Hoovered And Cleaned With Disinfectant										
14	Clean And Polish Bookshelves, Remember To Dust The Top										
15	Remove, Wash And Clean Any Dirty Cups Or Glasses										
16	Remove, Wash And Clean Any Dirty Plates, Bowels Or Cutlery										
17	Clean And Sanitize Any Chairs And Seats										
18	Water Jug (Washed Thoroughly Each Day & Re-Filled)										
19	Water Any Plants And Flowers										
20	Dust Plant Leafs (A Healthy Plant Needs To Be Clear Of Dust)										
21	Empty The Waste Basket And Recycling Bin										
22	Clean And Disinfectant The Waste Bin And Recycling Bin										
23	Clean And Wipe Down Windowsills										
24	Spray Air Freshener This Keeps The Room Smelling Fresh										
25	Clean And Disinfect Cabinets And Units										
26	Clean And Sanitize Desk Accessories										
27	Replace Dirty Linen And Move To Laundry Room										
28	Polish Any Wooden Furniture And Hardwood Surfaces										
29	Clean Skirting Boards/Baseboards And Corners										

Care Home Cleaning Tasks - Bedrooms Continued	M	T	W	T	F	S	S	Cleaned By	Checked By	Date/Time
Dust Television, Top Sides And Back, TV Unit And TV Stand										
Clean TV Screen With Soft Damp Cloth (Use Water/Cleaner)										
Vacuum/Hoover Between Bedroom Furniture And The Walls										
Clean And Sanitize Resident's Personal Wheelchair										
Check For Broken Wheelchairs, Frames and Wheels										
Vacuum Under Furniture, Beds, Sofas and Dressers										
Vacuum And Hoover The Carpets, Mats And Rugs										
Vacuum Furnishings, Cushions, Chairs, Sofas And Couches										
Steam Clean Carpets And Rugs										
Dust And Clean Any Picture Frames And Photo Frames										
Ledges, Flat Surfaces And The Tops Of Wardrobes Dusted										
Clean & Check Contents Of Medicine Trolleys & Cupboards										
Clean And Sanitize Mobile Phone, Phone Case And Screen										
Clean & Vacuum The Desk Chair, Legs And Chair Wheels										
Wash And Clean Air Vents										
Dust Ceiling Fan Blades With Duster Or A Microfibre Cloth										
Wash And Clean Windows (Inside And Outside)										
Dust And Clean The Walls From Top To Bottom										
Clean Blinds (Dust The Blinds With A Damp Microfibre Cloth)										
Clean Curtains (Vacuum On A Low Setting Or Wash If Possible)										
Dust And Wash Radiator Covers										
Wash And Clean Ceiling Light Covers										
Clean & Vacuum Central Heating Units (Backs Of Radiators)										
Clean And Disinfect Any Handrails										
Hand Towels Replaced With Fresh Clean Ones										
Sink Wall Mirror Cleaned With Glass Cleaner										
Sinks, Taps And Fixtures Cleaned And Disinfected										
Pour Drain Cleaner Down Sink Drains										
Check For Broken Furniture (Report/Schedule Maintenance)										
Light Bulbs Checked And None Functioning Bulbs Replaced										
Check Hardware, Door Stops And Lock Mechanisms										
Fire Exit Lights And Emergency Lights Checked & Functioning										
Test Carbon Monoxide Alarm And Replace Batteries If Required										
Test Smoke Detector Alarm And Replace Batteries If Required										
Paper Dispensers And Paper Towel Rolls Re-Stocked										
Soap Dispensers, Hand Sanitizers And Hand Gels Are Refilled										
Face Masks, Protective Gloves And Face Shields Re-Stocked										

CARE HOME COMMUNAL AREA CLEANING *Checklist*

Building	Location	Room Number	Area

Start Date & Time	Finnish Date & Time	Name	Signature

	Care Home Cleaning Tasks - Communal Area	M	T	W	T	F	S	S	Cleaned By	Checked By	Date/Tim
1	Clean And Sanitize All The Desks And Tables										
2	Clean And Sanitize All The Counter Tops And Surface Areas										
3	Wipe Down The Walls Wherever There Are Spills And Splashes										
4	Disinfect Touch Points, Light Switches And Other Switches										
5	Clean And Disinfect All Doors, Handles And Doorknobs										
6	Clean And Dust Door Frames, Remember To Dust The Tops										
7	Dust Light Fixtures & Shades With A Duster Or A Microfibre Cloth										
8	Clean And Wipe Mirrors Remove Fingerprints, Smears & Dirt										
9	Clean And Sanitize Over Chair Tables										
10	Clean And Polish Bookshelves, Remember To Dust The Top										
11	Remove, Wash And Clean Any Dirty Cups Or Glasses										
12	Remove, Wash And Clean Any Dirty Plates, Bowels Or Cutlery										
13	Clean And Sanitize Any Chairs, Seats And Benches										
14	Water Jugs (Washed Thoroughly Each Day & Re-Filled)										
15	Water Any Plants And Flowers										
16	Dust Plant Leafs (A Healthy Plant Needs To Be Clear Of Dust)										
17	Empty The Waste Baskets And Recycling Bins										
18	Clean And Disinfectant The Waste Bins And Recycling Bins										
19	Clean And Wipe Down Windowsills										
20	Spray Air Freshener This Keeps The Room Smelling Fresh										
21	Clean And Disinfect Cabinets And Units										
22	Clean And Sanitize Desk Accessories										
23	Replace Dirty Table Linen And Move To Laundry Room										
24	Polish Any Wooden Furniture And Hardwood Surfaces										
25	Clean Skirting Boards/Baseboards And Corners										
26	Clean And Polish Fireplace Mantelpiece And Surrounds										
27	Wipe Down Equipment & Sanitize Tea And Coffee Making Facilities										
28	Clean And Sanitize Telephones, Cords/Leads & All Touch Points										
29	Clean And Sanitize Walking Sticks And Any Other Walking Aids										

Care Home Cleaning Tasks - Communal Area	M	T	W	T	F	S	S	Cleaned By	Checked By	Date/Time
Dust Television, Top Sides And Back, TV Unit And TV Stand										
Clean TV Screen With Soft Damp Cloth (Use Water/Cleaner)										
Vacuum/Hoover Between Furniture And The Walls										
Clean And Sanitize All Wheelchairs										
Check For Broken Wheelchairs, Frames and Wheels										
Vacuum Under Furniture, Units, Tables And Cabinets										
Vacuum And Hoover The Carpets, Mats And Rugs										
Vacuum Furnishings, Cushions, Chairs, Sofas And Couches										
Steam Clean Carpets And Rugs										
Dust And Clean Any Picture Frames And Wall Art										
Clean & Check Contents Of Medicine Trolleys & Cupboards										
Clean & Vacuum The Desk Chair, Legs And Chair Wheels										
Wash And Clean Air Vents										
Dust Ceiling Fan Blades With Duster Or A Microfibre Cloth										
Wash And Clean Windows (Inside And Outside)										
Dust And Clean The Walls From Top To Bottom										
Clean Blinds (Dust The Blinds With A Damp Microfibre Cloth)										
Clean Curtains (Vacuum On A Low Setting Or Wash If Possible)										
Dust And Wash Radiator Covers										
Wash And Clean Ceiling Light Covers										
Clean & Vacuum Central Heating Units (Backs Of Radiators)										
Clean And Disinfect Any Handrails										
Clean And Sanitize Computer, Keyboard And Computer Mice										
Clean And Sanitize iPads, Tablets, Laptops & Mobile Phones										
Floors Mopped Clean With Cleaning Or Disinfecting Solution										
The Floors Are Swept And Free From Debris And Litter										
Clean Sliding Doors and Room Partitions										
Throw Away Outdated Newspapers, Magazines, Papers										
Check For Broken Furniture (Report/Schedule Maintenance)										
Light Bulbs Checked And None Functioning Bulbs Replaced										
Check Hardware, Door Stops And Lock Mechanisms										
Fire Exit Lights And Emergency Lights Checked & Functioning										
Test Carbon Monoxide Alarm And Replace Batteries If Required										
Test Smoke Detector Alarm And Replace Batteries If Required										
Paper Dispensers And Paper Towel Rolls Re-Stocked										
Soap Dispensers, Hand Sanitizers And Hand Gels Are Refilled										
Face Masks, Protective Gloves And Face Shields Re-Stocked										

CARE HOME TOILET & RESTROOM CLEANING *Checklist*

Building	Location	Room Number	Area

Start Date & Time	Finnish Date & Time	Name	Signature

	Care Home Cleaning Tasks - Toilet & Restroom	M	T	W	T	F	S	S	Cleaned By	Checked By	Date/Time
1	Clean And Sanitize All The Counter Tops And Surface Areas										
2	Wipe Down The Walls Wherever There Are Spills And Splashes										
3	Disinfect Touch Points, Light Switches And Other Switches										
4	Clean And Disinfect All Doors, Handles And Doorknobs										
5	Clean And Dust Door Frames, Remember To Dust The Tops										
6	Dust Light Fixtures With A Duster Or A Microfibre Cloth										
7	Wall Mirrors Cleaned With Glass Cleaner										
8	Clean Any Bathroom Glasses And Cups										
9	Clean And Sanitize Any Chairs And Seats										
10	Empty The Waste Basket And Recycling Bin										
11	Clean And Disinfectant The Waste Bin And Recycling Bin										
12	Clean And Wipe Down Windowsills										
13	Spray Air Freshener This Keeps The Room Smelling Fresh										
14	Air/Odour Control Systems Are Filled And Operating Correctly										
15	Clean Skirting Boards/Baseboards And Corners										
16	Vacuum And Hoover Bath Mats, Shower Mats And Rugs										
17	Replace Bath Mats, Shower Mats And Rugs With Clean Ones										
18	Steam Clean Carpets And Rugs										
19	Hand Towels Replaced With Fresh Clean Ones										
20	Bath Towels Replaced With Fresh Clean Ones										
21	Face Towels Replaced With Fresh Clean Ones										
22	Electric Hand Dryers Cleaned, Disinfected & Operating Correctly										
23	Soap Dispensers, Sanitizers And Hand Gels Are Refilled										
24	Clean & Check Contents Of Medicine Trolleys & Cupboards										
25	Clean And Disinfect Any Handrails										
26	Sinks, Taps And Fixtures Cleaned And Disinfected										
27	Clean And Disinfect Cabinets And Units										
28	Feminine Hygiene Dispensers Re-Stocked										
29	Feminine Hygiene Bins/Containers Emptied And Cleared										

Care Home Cleaning Tasks - Toilet & Restroom	M	T	W	T	F	S	S	Cleaned By	Checked By	Date/Time
Clean & Vacuum Central Heating Units (Backs Of Radiators)										
Wash And Clean Ceiling Light Covers										
Toilet Roll Holders And Toilet Rolls Re-Stocked										
Toilet Roll Holders Cleaned And Disinfected										
Clean Inside The Toilets And Urinals With Disinfectant										
Toilet Seats Cleaned And Disinfected										
Clean Top Of Toilets Tanks, The Bases And Behind Toilets										
Urinal Handles Cleaned And Disinfected										
Urinal Screens Cleaned, Disinfected And Blocks Replaced										
Paper Dispensers And Paper Towel Rolls Re-Stocked										
Paper Dispensers And Paper Towel Roll Cleaned & Disinfected										
The Floors Are Swept And Free From Debris And Litter										
Floors Mopped Clean With Cleaning Or Disinfecting Solution										
Put Up Or Place Wet Floor Signs After Mopping Floors										
Showers And Shower Heads, Cleaned And Disinfected										
Soak Shower Heads										
Clean And Disinfect Glass Shower Doors/Outer Doors										
Clean Soap Scum From Shower Walls										
Clean Blinds (Dust The Blinds With A Damp Microfibre Cloth)										
Clean Curtains (Vacuum On A Low Setting Or Wash If Possible)										
Dust And Wash Radiator Covers										
Clean And Disinfect Commodes Between Each Use										
Clean And Disinfect Shower Chairs Between Each Use										
Bath Hoists Cleaned And Disinfected Between Each Use										
Scrub Tub/Bath, Polish Facets And Taps, Clean & Disinfected										
Toothbrush Holders And Soap Holders Cleaned										
Re-Place Shower Curtains With Clean Fresh Ones										
Wash And Clean Air Vents										
Thoroughly Clean Grout And Tiles										
Disinfect And Clean All The Walls From Top To Bottom										
Wash And Clean Windows (Inside And Outside)										
Unclog The Drains (Sink, Bath And Shower)										
Pour Drain Cleaner Down Sink, Shower & Bath Drains										
Floor Drains And Drain Covers Are Open And Free Of Debris										
Hair Dryers Cleaned And Disinfected And Operating Correctly										
Light Bulbs Checked And None Functioning Bulbs Replaced										
Check Hardware, Door Stops And Lock Mechanisms										

CARE HOME BEDROOM CLEANING *Checklist*

Building	Location	Room Number	Area

Start Date & Time	Finnish Date & Time	Name	Signature

	Care Home Cleaning Tasks - Bedrooms	M	T	W	T	F	S	S	Cleaned By	Checked By	Date/Tim
1	Clean And Sanitize All The Desks And Tables										
2	Clean And Sanitize All The Counter Tops And Surface Areas										
3	Wipe Down The Walls Wherever There Are Spills And Splashes										
4	Disinfect Touch Points, Light Switches And Other Switches										
5	Clean And Disinfect All Doors, Handles And Doorknobs										
6	Clean And Dust Door Frames, Remember To Dust The Tops										
7	Dust Light Fixtures With A Duster Or A Microfibre Cloth										
8	Clean & Wipe Mirrors Remove Fingerprints, Smears & Dirt										
9	Clean And Dust Bedside Cabinets										
10	Clean And Sanitize Over Chair Tables										
11	Clean And Sanitize Over Bed Tables										
12	Clean And Check Bed Frames										
13	Mattresses Hoovered And Cleaned With Disinfectant										
14	Clean And Polish Bookshelves, Remember To Dust The Top										
15	Remove, Wash And Clean Any Dirty Cups Or Glasses										
16	Remove, Wash And Clean Any Dirty Plates, Bowels Or Cutlery										
17	Clean And Sanitize Any Chairs And Seats										
18	Water Jug (Washed Thoroughly Each Day & Re-Filled)										
19	Water Any Plants And Flowers										
20	Dust Plant Leafs (A Healthy Plant Needs To Be Clear Of Dust)										
21	Empty The Waste Basket And Recycling Bin										
22	Clean And Disinfectant The Waste Bin And Recycling Bin										
23	Clean And Wipe Down Windowsills										
24	Spray Air Freshener This Keeps The Room Smelling Fresh										
25	Clean And Disinfect Cabinets And Units										
26	Clean And Sanitize Desk Accessories										
27	Replace Dirty Linen And Move To Laundry Room										
28	Polish Any Wooden Furniture And Hardwood Surfaces										
29	Clean Skirting Boards/Baseboards And Corners										

Care Home Cleaning Tasks - Bedrooms Continued	M	T	W	T	F	S	S	Cleaned By	Checked By	Date/Time
Dust Television, Top Sides And Back, TV Unit And TV Stand										
Clean TV Screen With Soft Damp Cloth (Use Water/Cleaner)										
Vacuum/Hoover Between Bedroom Furniture And The Walls										
Clean And Sanitize Resident's Personal Wheelchair										
Check For Broken Wheelchairs, Frames and Wheels										
Vacuum Under Furniture, Beds, Sofas and Dressers										
Vacuum And Hoover The Carpets, Mats And Rugs										
Vacuum Furnishings, Cushions, Chairs, Sofas And Couches										
Steam Clean Carpets And Rugs										
Dust And Clean Any Picture Frames And Photo Frames										
Ledges, Flat Surfaces And The Tops Of Wardrobes Dusted										
Clean & Check Contents Of Medicine Trolleys & Cupboards										
Clean And Sanitize Mobile Phone, Phone Case And Screen										
Clean & Vacuum The Desk Chair, Legs And Chair Wheels										
Wash And Clean Air Vents										
Dust Ceiling Fan Blades With Duster Or A Microfibre Cloth										
Wash And Clean Windows (Inside And Outside)										
Dust And Clean The Walls From Top To Bottom										
Clean Blinds (Dust The Blinds With A Damp Microfibre Cloth)										
Clean Curtains (Vacuum On A Low Setting Or Wash If Possible)										
Dust And Wash Radiator Covers										
Wash And Clean Ceiling Light Covers										
Clean & Vacuum Central Heating Units (Backs Of Radiators)										
Clean And Disinfect Any Handrails										
Hand Towels Replaced With Fresh Clean Ones										
Sink Wall Mirror Cleaned With Glass Cleaner										
Sinks, Taps And Fixtures Cleaned And Disinfected										
Pour Drain Cleaner Down Sink Drains										
Check For Broken Furniture (Report/Schedule Maintenance)										
Light Bulbs Checked And None Functioning Bulbs Replaced										
Check Hardware, Door Stops And Lock Mechanisms										
Fire Exit Lights And Emergency Lights Checked & Functioning										
Test Carbon Monoxide Alarm And Replace Batteries If Required										
Test Smoke Detector Alarm And Replace Batteries If Required										
Paper Dispensers And Paper Towel Rolls Re-Stocked										
Soap Dispensers, Hand Sanitizers And Hand Gels Are Refilled										
Face Masks, Protective Gloves And Face Shields Re-Stocked										

CARE HOME COMMUNAL AREA CLEANING *Checklist*

Building	Location	Room Number	Area

Start Date & Time	Finnish Date & Time	Name	Signature

	Care Home Cleaning Tasks - Communal Area	M	T	W	T	F	S	S	Cleaned By	Checked By	Date/Tim
1	Clean And Sanitize All The Desks And Tables										
2	Clean And Sanitize All The Counter Tops And Surface Areas										
3	Wipe Down The Walls Wherever There Are Spills And Splashes										
4	Disinfect Touch Points, Light Switches And Other Switches										
5	Clean And Disinfect All Doors, Handles And Doorknobs										
6	Clean And Dust Door Frames, Remember To Dust The Tops										
7	Dust Light Fixtures & Shades With A Duster Or A Microfibre Cloth										
8	Clean And Wipe Mirrors Remove Fingerprints, Smears & Dirt										
9	Clean And Sanitize Over Chair Tables										
10	Clean And Polish Bookshelves, Remember To Dust The Top										
11	Remove, Wash And Clean Any Dirty Cups Or Glasses										
12	Remove, Wash And Clean Any Dirty Plates, Bowels Or Cutlery										
13	Clean And Sanitize Any Chairs, Seats And Benches										
14	Water Jugs (Washed Thoroughly Each Day & Re-Filled)										
15	Water Any Plants And Flowers										
16	Dust Plant Leafs (A Healthy Plant Needs To Be Clear Of Dust)										
17	Empty The Waste Baskets And Recycling Bins										
18	Clean And Disinfectant The Waste Bins And Recycling Bins										
19	Clean And Wipe Down Windowsills										
20	Spray Air Freshener This Keeps The Room Smelling Fresh										
21	Clean And Disinfect Cabinets And Units										
22	Clean And Sanitize Desk Accessories										
23	Replace Dirty Table Linen And Move To Laundry Room										
24	Polish Any Wooden Furniture And Hardwood Surfaces										
25	Clean Skirting Boards/Baseboards And Corners										
26	Clean And Polish Fireplace Mantelpiece And Surrounds										
27	Wipe Down Equipment & Sanitize Tea And Coffee Making Facilities										
28	Clean And Sanitize Telephones, Cords/Leads & All Touch Points										
29	Clean And Sanitize Walking Sticks And Any Other Walking Aids										

Care Home Cleaning Tasks - Communal Area	M	T	W	T	F	S	S	Cleaned By	Checked By	Date/Time
Dust Television, Top Sides And Back, TV Unit And TV Stand										
Clean TV Screen With Soft Damp Cloth (Use Water/Cleaner)										
Vacuum/Hoover Between Furniture And The Walls										
Clean And Sanitize All Wheelchairs										
Check For Broken Wheelchairs, Frames and Wheels										
Vacuum Under Furniture, Units, Tables And Cabinets										
Vacuum And Hoover The Carpets, Mats And Rugs										
Vacuum Furnishings, Cushions, Chairs, Sofas And Couches										
Steam Clean Carpets And Rugs										
Dust And Clean Any Picture Frames And Wall Art										
Clean & Check Contents Of Medicine Trolleys & Cupboards										
Clean & Vacuum The Desk Chair, Legs And Chair Wheels										
Wash And Clean Air Vents										
Dust Ceiling Fan Blades With Duster Or A Microfibre Cloth										
Wash And Clean Windows (Inside And Outside)										
Dust And Clean The Walls From Top To Bottom										
Clean Blinds (Dust The Blinds With A Damp Microfibre Cloth)										
Clean Curtains (Vacuum On A Low Setting Or Wash If Possible)										
Dust And Wash Radiator Covers										
Wash And Clean Ceiling Light Covers										
Clean & Vacuum Central Heating Units (Backs Of Radiators)										
Clean And Disinfect Any Handrails										
Clean And Sanitize Computer, Keyboard And Computer Mice										
Clean And Sanitize iPads, Tablets, Laptops & Mobile Phones										
Floors Mopped Clean With Cleaning Or Disinfecting Solution										
The Floors Are Swept And Free From Debris And Litter										
Clean Sliding Doors and Room Partitions										
Throw Away Outdated Newspapers, Magazines, Papers										
Check For Broken Furniture (Report/Schedule Maintenance)										
Light Bulbs Checked And None Functioning Bulbs Replaced										
Check Hardware, Door Stops And Lock Mechanisms										
Fire Exit Lights And Emergency Lights Checked & Functioning										
Test Carbon Monoxide Alarm And Replace Batteries If Required										
Test Smoke Detector Alarm And Replace Batteries If Required										
Paper Dispensers And Paper Towel Rolls Re-Stocked										
Soap Dispensers, Hand Sanitizers And Hand Gels Are Refilled										
Face Masks, Protective Gloves And Face Shields Re-Stocked										

CARE HOME TOILET & RESTROOM CLEANING *Checklist*

Building	Location	Room Number	Area

Start Date & Time	Finnish Date & Time	Name	Signature

	Care Home Cleaning Tasks - Toilet & Restroom	M	T	W	T	F	S	S	Cleaned By	Checked By	Date/Tim
1	Clean And Sanitize All The Counter Tops And Surface Areas										
2	Wipe Down The Walls Wherever There Are Spills And Splashes										
3	Disinfect Touch Points, Light Switches And Other Switches										
4	Clean And Disinfect All Doors, Handles And Doorknobs										
5	Clean And Dust Door Frames, Remember To Dust The Tops										
6	Dust Light Fixtures With A Duster Or A Microfibre Cloth										
7	Wall Mirrors Cleaned With Glass Cleaner										
8	Clean Any Bathroom Glasses And Cups										
9	Clean And Sanitize Any Chairs And Seats										
10	Empty The Waste Basket And Recycling Bin										
11	Clean And Disinfectant The Waste Bin And Recycling Bin										
12	Clean And Wipe Down Windowsills										
13	Spray Air Freshener This Keeps The Room Smelling Fresh										
14	Air/Odour Control Systems Are Filled And Operating Correctly										
15	Clean Skirting Boards/Baseboards And Corners										
16	Vacuum And Hoover Bath Mats, Shower Mats And Rugs										
17	Replace Bath Mats, Shower Mats And Rugs With Clean Ones										
18	Steam Clean Carpets And Rugs										
19	Hand Towels Replaced With Fresh Clean Ones										
20	Bath Towels Replaced With Fresh Clean Ones										
21	Face Towels Replaced With Fresh Clean Ones										
22	Electric Hand Dryers Cleaned, Disinfected & Operating Correctly										
23	Soap Dispensers, Sanitizers And Hand Gels Are Refilled										
24	Clean & Check Contents Of Medicine Trolleys & Cupboards										
25	Clean And Disinfect Any Handrails										
26	Sinks, Taps And Fixtures Cleaned And Disinfected										
27	Clean And Disinfect Cabinets And Units										
28	Feminine Hygiene Dispensers Re-Stocked										
29	Feminine Hygiene Bins/Containers Emptied And Cleared										

Care Home Cleaning Tasks - Toilet & Restroom	M	T	W	T	F	S	S	Cleaned By	Checked By	Date/Time
Clean & Vacuum Central Heating Units (Backs Of Radiators)										
Wash And Clean Ceiling Light Covers										
Toilet Roll Holders And Toilet Rolls Re-Stocked										
Toilet Roll Holders Cleaned And Disinfected										
Clean Inside The Toilets And Urinals With Disinfectant										
Toilet Seats Cleaned And Disinfected										
Clean Top Of Toilets Tanks, The Bases And Behind Toilets										
Urinal Handles Cleaned And Disinfected										
Urinal Screens Cleaned, Disinfected And Blocks Replaced										
Paper Dispensers And Paper Towel Rolls Re-Stocked										
Paper Dispensers And Paper Towel Roll Cleaned & Disinfected										
The Floors Are Swept And Free From Debris And Litter										
Floors Mopped Clean With Cleaning Or Disinfecting Solution										
Put Up Or Place Wet Floor Signs After Mopping Floors										
Showers And Shower Heads, Cleaned And Disinfected										
Soak Shower Heads										
Clean And Disinfect Glass Shower Doors/Outer Doors										
Clean Soap Scum From Shower Walls										
Clean Blinds (Dust The Blinds With A Damp Microfibre Cloth)										
Clean Curtains (Vacuum On A Low Setting Or Wash If Possible)										
Dust And Wash Radiator Covers										
Clean And Disinfect Commodes Between Each Use										
Clean And Disinfect Shower Chairs Between Each Use										
Bath Hoists Cleaned And Disinfected Between Each Use										
Scrub Tub/Bath, Polish Facets And Taps, Clean & Disinfected										
Toothbrush Holders And Soap Holders Cleaned										
Re-Place Shower Curtains With Clean Fresh Ones										
Wash And Clean Air Vents										
Thoroughly Clean Grout And Tiles										
Disinfect And Clean All The Walls From Top To Bottom										
Wash And Clean Windows (Inside And Outside)										
Unclog The Drains (Sink, Bath And Shower)										
Pour Drain Cleaner Down Sink, Shower & Bath Drains										
Floor Drains And Drain Covers Are Open And Free Of Debris										
Hair Dryers Cleaned And Disinfected And Operating Correctly										
Light Bulbs Checked And None Functioning Bulbs Replaced										
Check Hardware, Door Stops And Lock Mechanisms										

CARE HOME BEDROOM CLEANING *Checklist*

Building	Location	Room Number	Area

Start Date & Time	Finnish Date & Time	Name	Signature

	Care Home Cleaning Tasks - Bedrooms	M	T	W	T	F	S	S	Cleaned By	Checked By	Date/Tir
1	Clean And Sanitize All The Desks And Tables										
2	Clean And Sanitize All The Counter Tops And Surface Areas										
3	Wipe Down The Walls Wherever There Are Spills And Splashes										
4	Disinfect Touch Points, Light Switches And Other Switches										
5	Clean And Disinfect All Doors, Handles And Doorknobs										
6	Clean And Dust Door Frames, Remember To Dust The Tops										
7	Dust Light Fixtures With A Duster Or A Microfibre Cloth										
8	Clean & Wipe Mirrors Remove Fingerprints, Smears & Dirt										
9	Clean And Dust Bedside Cabinets										
10	Clean And Sanitize Over Chair Tables										
11	Clean And Sanitize Over Bed Tables										
12	Clean And Check Bed Frames										
13	Mattresses Hoovered And Cleaned With Disinfectant										
14	Clean And Polish Bookshelves, Remember To Dust The Top										
15	Remove, Wash And Clean Any Dirty Cups Or Glasses										
16	Remove, Wash And Clean Any Dirty Plates, Bowels Or Cutlery										
17	Clean And Sanitize Any Chairs And Seats										
18	Water Jug (Washed Thoroughly Each Day & Re-Filled)										
19	Water Any Plants And Flowers										
20	Dust Plant Leafs (A Healthy Plant Needs To Be Clear Of Dust)										
21	Empty The Waste Basket And Recycling Bin										
22	Clean And Disinfectant The Waste Bin And Recycling Bin										
23	Clean And Wipe Down Windowsills										
24	Spray Air Freshener This Keeps The Room Smelling Fresh										
25	Clean And Disinfect Cabinets And Units										
26	Clean And Sanitize Desk Accessories										
27	Replace Dirty Linen And Move To Laundry Room										
28	Polish Any Wooden Furniture And Hardwood Surfaces										
29	Clean Skirting Boards/Baseboards And Corners										

Care Home Cleaning Tasks - Bedrooms Continued	M	T	W	T	F	S	S	Cleaned By	Checked By	Date/Time
Dust Television, Top Sides And Back, TV Unit And TV Stand										
Clean TV Screen With Soft Damp Cloth (Use Water/Cleaner)										
Vacuum/Hoover Between Bedroom Furniture And The Walls										
Clean And Sanitize Resident's Personal Wheelchair										
Check For Broken Wheelchairs, Frames and Wheels										
Vacuum Under Furniture, Beds, Sofas and Dressers										
Vacuum And Hoover The Carpets, Mats And Rugs										
Vacuum Furnishings, Cushions, Chairs, Sofas And Couches										
Steam Clean Carpets And Rugs										
Dust And Clean Any Picture Frames And Photo Frames										
Ledges, Flat Surfaces And The Tops Of Wardrobes Dusted										
Clean & Check Contents Of Medicine Trolleys & Cupboards										
Clean And Sanitize Mobile Phone, Phone Case And Screen										
Clean & Vacuum The Desk Chair, Legs And Chair Wheels										
Wash And Clean Air Vents										
Dust Ceiling Fan Blades With Duster Or A Microfibre Cloth										
Wash And Clean Windows (Inside And Outside)										
Dust And Clean The Walls From Top To Bottom										
Clean Blinds (Dust The Blinds With A Damp Microfibre Cloth)										
Clean Curtains (Vacuum On A Low Setting Or Wash If Possible)										
Dust And Wash Radiator Covers										
Wash And Clean Ceiling Light Covers										
Clean & Vacuum Central Heating Units (Backs Of Radiators)										
Clean And Disinfect Any Handrails										
Hand Towels Replaced With Fresh Clean Ones										
Sink Wall Mirror Cleaned With Glass Cleaner										
Sinks, Taps And Fixtures Cleaned And Disinfected										
Pour Drain Cleaner Down Sink Drains										
Check For Broken Furniture (Report/Schedule Maintenance)										
Light Bulbs Checked And None Functioning Bulbs Replaced										
Check Hardware, Door Stops And Lock Mechanisms										
Fire Exit Lights And Emergency Lights Checked & Functioning										
Test Carbon Monoxide Alarm And Replace Batteries If Required										
Test Smoke Detector Alarm And Replace Batteries If Required										
Paper Dispensers And Paper Towel Rolls Re-Stocked										
Soap Dispensers, Hand Sanitizers And Hand Gels Are Refilled										
Face Masks, Protective Gloves And Face Shields Re-Stocked										

CARE HOME COMMUNAL AREA CLEANING *Checklist*

Building	Location	Room Number	Area

Start Date & Time	Finnish Date & Time	Name	Signature

	Care Home Cleaning Tasks - Communal Area	M	T	W	T	F	S	S	Cleaned By	Checked By	Date/Tim
1	Clean And Sanitize All The Desks And Tables										
2	Clean And Sanitize All The Counter Tops And Surface Areas										
3	Wipe Down The Walls Wherever There Are Spills And Splashes										
4	Disinfect Touch Points, Light Switches And Other Switches										
5	Clean And Disinfect All Doors, Handles And Doorknobs										
6	Clean And Dust Door Frames, Remember To Dust The Tops										
7	Dust Light Fixtures & Shades With A Duster Or A Microfibre Cloth										
8	Clean And Wipe Mirrors Remove Fingerprints, Smears & Dirt										
9	Clean And Sanitize Over Chair Tables										
10	Clean And Polish Bookshelves, Remember To Dust The Top										
11	Remove, Wash And Clean Any Dirty Cups Or Glasses										
12	Remove, Wash And Clean Any Dirty Plates, Bowels Or Cutlery										
13	Clean And Sanitize Any Chairs, Seats And Benches										
14	Water Jugs (Washed Thoroughly Each Day & Re-Filled)										
15	Water Any Plants And Flowers										
16	Dust Plant Leafs (A Healthy Plant Needs To Be Clear Of Dust)										
17	Empty The Waste Baskets And Recycling Bins										
18	Clean And Disinfectant The Waste Bins And Recycling Bins										
19	Clean And Wipe Down Windowsills										
20	Spray Air Freshener This Keeps The Room Smelling Fresh										
21	Clean And Disinfect Cabinets And Units										
22	Clean And Sanitize Desk Accessories										
23	Replace Dirty Table Linen And Move To Laundry Room										
24	Polish Any Wooden Furniture And Hardwood Surfaces										
25	Clean Skirting Boards/Baseboards And Corners										
26	Clean And Polish Fireplace Mantelpiece And Surrounds										
27	Wipe Down Equipment & Sanitize Tea And Coffee Making Facilities										
28	Clean And Sanitize Telephones, Cords/Leads & All Touch Points										
29	Clean And Sanitize Walking Sticks And Any Other Walking Aids										

Care Home Cleaning Tasks - Communal Area	M	T	W	T	F	S	S	Cleaned By	Checked By	Date/Time
Dust Television, Top Sides And Back, TV Unit And TV Stand										
Clean TV Screen With Soft Damp Cloth (Use Water/Cleaner)										
Vacuum/Hoover Between Furniture And The Walls										
Clean And Sanitize All Wheelchairs										
Check For Broken Wheelchairs, Frames and Wheels										
Vacuum Under Furniture, Units, Tables And Cabinets										
Vacuum And Hoover The Carpets, Mats And Rugs										
Vacuum Furnishings, Cushions, Chairs, Sofas And Couches										
Steam Clean Carpets And Rugs										
Dust And Clean Any Picture Frames And Wall Art										
Clean & Check Contents Of Medicine Trolleys & Cupboards										
Clean & Vacuum The Desk Chair, Legs And Chair Wheels										
Wash And Clean Air Vents										
Dust Ceiling Fan Blades With Duster Or A Microfibre Cloth										
Wash And Clean Windows (Inside And Outside)										
Dust And Clean The Walls From Top To Bottom										
Clean Blinds (Dust The Blinds With A Damp Microfibre Cloth)										
Clean Curtains (Vacuum On A Low Setting Or Wash If Possible)										
Dust And Wash Radiator Covers										
Wash And Clean Ceiling Light Covers										
Clean & Vacuum Central Heating Units (Backs Of Radiators)										
Clean And Disinfect Any Handrails										
Clean And Sanitize Computer, Keyboard And Computer Mice										
Clean And Sanitize iPads, Tablets, Laptops & Mobile Phones										
Floors Mopped Clean With Cleaning Or Disinfecting Solution										
The Floors Are Swept And Free From Debris And Litter										
Clean Sliding Doors and Room Partitions										
Throw Away Outdated Newspapers, Magazines, Papers										
Check For Broken Furniture (Report/Schedule Maintenance)										
Light Bulbs Checked And None Functioning Bulbs Replaced										
Check Hardware, Door Stops And Lock Mechanisms										
Fire Exit Lights And Emergency Lights Checked & Functioning										
Test Carbon Monoxide Alarm And Replace Batteries If Required										
Test Smoke Detector Alarm And Replace Batteries If Required										
Paper Dispensers And Paper Towel Rolls Re-Stocked										
Soap Dispensers, Hand Sanitizers And Hand Gels Are Refilled										
Face Masks, Protective Gloves And Face Shields Re-Stocked										

CARE HOME TOILET & RESTROOM CLEANING *Checklist*

Building	Location	Room Number	Area

Start Date & Time	Finnish Date & Time	Name	Signature

	Care Home Cleaning Tasks - Toilet & Restroom	M	T	W	T	F	S	S	Cleaned By	Checked By	Date/Tim
1	Clean And Sanitize All The Counter Tops And Surface Areas										
2	Wipe Down The Walls Wherever There Are Spills And Splashes										
3	Disinfect Touch Points, Light Switches And Other Switches										
4	Clean And Disinfect All Doors, Handles And Doorknobs										
5	Clean And Dust Door Frames, Remember To Dust The Tops										
6	Dust Light Fixtures With A Duster Or A Microfibre Cloth										
7	Wall Mirrors Cleaned With Glass Cleaner										
8	Clean Any Bathroom Glasses And Cups										
9	Clean And Sanitize Any Chairs And Seats										
10	Empty The Waste Basket And Recycling Bin										
11	Clean And Disinfectant The Waste Bin And Recycling Bin										
12	Clean And Wipe Down Windowsills										
13	Spray Air Freshener This Keeps The Room Smelling Fresh										
14	Air/Odour Control Systems Are Filled And Operating Correctly										
15	Clean Skirting Boards/Baseboards And Corners										
16	Vacuum And Hoover Bath Mats, Shower Mats And Rugs										
17	Replace Bath Mats, Shower Mats And Rugs With Clean Ones										
18	Steam Clean Carpets And Rugs										
19	Hand Towels Replaced With Fresh Clean Ones										
20	Bath Towels Replaced With Fresh Clean Ones										
21	Face Towels Replaced With Fresh Clean Ones										
22	Electric Hand Dryers Cleaned, Disinfected & Operating Correctly										
23	Soap Dispensers, Sanitizers And Hand Gels Are Refilled										
24	Clean & Check Contents Of Medicine Trolleys & Cupboards										
25	Clean And Disinfect Any Handrails										
26	Sinks, Taps And Fixtures Cleaned And Disinfected										
27	Clean And Disinfect Cabinets And Units										
28	Feminine Hygiene Dispensers Re-Stocked										
29	Feminine Hygiene Bins/Containers Emptied And Cleared										

Care Home Cleaning Tasks - Toilet & Restroom	M	T	W	T	F	S	S	Cleaned By	Checked By	Date/Time
Clean & Vacuum Central Heating Units (Backs Of Radiators)										
Wash And Clean Ceiling Light Covers										
Toilet Roll Holders And Toilet Rolls Re-Stocked										
Toilet Roll Holders Cleaned And Disinfected										
Clean Inside The Toilets And Urinals With Disinfectant										
Toilet Seats Cleaned And Disinfected										
Clean Top Of Toilets Tanks, The Bases And Behind Toilets										
Urinal Handles Cleaned And Disinfected										
Urinal Screens Cleaned, Disinfected And Blocks Replaced										
Paper Dispensers And Paper Towel Rolls Re-Stocked										
Paper Dispensers And Paper Towel Roll Cleaned & Disinfected										
The Floors Are Swept And Free From Debris And Litter										
Floors Mopped Clean With Cleaning Or Disinfecting Solution										
Put Up Or Place Wet Floor Signs After Mopping Floors										
Showers And Shower Heads, Cleaned And Disinfected										
Soak Shower Heads										
Clean And Disinfect Glass Shower Doors/Outer Doors										
Clean Soap Scum From Shower Walls										
Clean Blinds (Dust The Blinds With A Damp Microfibre Cloth)										
Clean Curtains (Vacuum On A Low Setting Or Wash If Possible)										
Dust And Wash Radiator Covers										
Clean And Disinfect Commodes Between Each Use										
Clean And Disinfect Shower Chairs Between Each Use										
Bath Hoists Cleaned And Disinfected Between Each Use										
Scrub Tub/Bath, Polish Facets And Taps, Clean & Disinfected										
Toothbrush Holders And Soap Holders Cleaned										
Re-Place Shower Curtains With Clean Fresh Ones										
Wash And Clean Air Vents										
Thoroughly Clean Grout And Tiles										
Disinfect And Clean All The Walls From Top To Bottom										
Wash And Clean Windows (Inside And Outside)										
Unclog The Drains (Sink, Bath And Shower)										
Pour Drain Cleaner Down Sink, Shower & Bath Drains										
Floor Drains And Drain Covers Are Open And Free Of Debris										
Hair Dryers Cleaned And Disinfected And Operating Correctly										
Light Bulbs Checked And None Functioning Bulbs Replaced										
Check Hardware, Door Stops And Lock Mechanisms										

CARE HOME BEDROOM CLEANING *Checklist*

Building	Location	Room Number	Area

Start Date & Time	Finnish Date & Time	Name	Signature

	Care Home Cleaning Tasks - Bedrooms	M	T	W	T	F	S	S	Cleaned By	Checked By	Date/Tim
1	Clean And Sanitize All The Desks And Tables										
2	Clean And Sanitize All The Counter Tops And Surface Areas										
3	Wipe Down The Walls Wherever There Are Spills And Splashes										
4	Disinfect Touch Points, Light Switches And Other Switches										
5	Clean And Disinfect All Doors, Handles And Doorknobs										
6	Clean And Dust Door Frames, Remember To Dust The Tops										
7	Dust Light Fixtures With A Duster Or A Microfibre Cloth										
8	Clean & Wipe Mirrors Remove Fingerprints, Smears & Dirt										
9	Clean And Dust Bedside Cabinets										
10	Clean And Sanitize Over Chair Tables										
11	Clean And Sanitize Over Bed Tables										
12	Clean And Check Bed Frames										
13	Mattresses Hoovered And Cleaned With Disinfectant										
14	Clean And Polish Bookshelves, Remember To Dust The Top										
15	Remove, Wash And Clean Any Dirty Cups Or Glasses										
16	Remove, Wash And Clean Any Dirty Plates, Bowels Or Cutlery										
17	Clean And Sanitize Any Chairs And Seats										
18	Water Jug (Washed Thoroughly Each Day & Re-Filled)										
19	Water Any Plants And Flowers										
20	Dust Plant Leafs (A Healthy Plant Needs To Be Clear Of Dust)										
21	Empty The Waste Basket And Recycling Bin										
22	Clean And Disinfectant The Waste Bin And Recycling Bin										
23	Clean And Wipe Down Windowsills										
24	Spray Air Freshener This Keeps The Room Smelling Fresh										
25	Clean And Disinfect Cabinets And Units										
26	Clean And Sanitize Desk Accessories										
27	Replace Dirty Linen And Move To Laundry Room										
28	Polish Any Wooden Furniture And Hardwood Surfaces										
29	Clean Skirting Boards/Baseboards And Corners										

Care Home Cleaning Tasks - Bedrooms Continued	M	T	W	T	F	S	S	Cleaned By	Checked By	Date/Time
Dust Television, Top Sides And Back, TV Unit And TV Stand										
Clean TV Screen With Soft Damp Cloth (Use Water/Cleaner)										
Vacuum/Hoover Between Bedroom Furniture And The Walls										
Clean And Sanitize Resident's Personal Wheelchair										
Check For Broken Wheelchairs, Frames and Wheels										
Vacuum Under Furniture, Beds, Sofas and Dressers										
Vacuum And Hoover The Carpets, Mats And Rugs										
Vacuum Furnishings, Cushions, Chairs, Sofas And Couches										
Steam Clean Carpets And Rugs										
Dust And Clean Any Picture Frames And Photo Frames										
Ledges, Flat Surfaces And The Tops Of Wardrobes Dusted										
Clean & Check Contents Of Medicine Trolleys & Cupboards										
Clean And Sanitize Mobile Phone, Phone Case And Screen										
Clean & Vacuum The Desk Chair, Legs And Chair Wheels										
Wash And Clean Air Vents										
Dust Ceiling Fan Blades With Duster Or A Microfibre Cloth										
Wash And Clean Windows (Inside And Outside)										
Dust And Clean The Walls From Top To Bottom										
Clean Blinds (Dust The Blinds With A Damp Microfibre Cloth)										
Clean Curtains (Vacuum On A Low Setting Or Wash If Possible)										
Dust And Wash Radiator Covers										
Wash And Clean Ceiling Light Covers										
Clean & Vacuum Central Heating Units (Backs Of Radiators)										
Clean And Disinfect Any Handrails										
Hand Towels Replaced With Fresh Clean Ones										
Sink Wall Mirror Cleaned With Glass Cleaner										
Sinks, Taps And Fixtures Cleaned And Disinfected										
Pour Drain Cleaner Down Sink Drains										
Check For Broken Furniture (Report/Schedule Maintenance)										
Light Bulbs Checked And None Functioning Bulbs Replaced										
Check Hardware, Door Stops And Lock Mechanisms										
Fire Exit Lights And Emergency Lights Checked & Functioning										
Test Carbon Monoxide Alarm And Replace Batteries If Required										
Test Smoke Detector Alarm And Replace Batteries If Required										
Paper Dispensers And Paper Towel Rolls Re-Stocked										
Soap Dispensers, Hand Sanitizers And Hand Gels Are Refilled										
Face Masks, Protective Gloves And Face Shields Re-Stocked										

CARE HOME COMMUNAL AREA CLEANING *Checklist*

Building	Location	Room Number	Area

Start Date & Time	Finnish Date & Time	Name	Signature

	Care Home Cleaning Tasks - Communal Area	M	T	W	T	F	S	S	Cleaned By	Checked By	Date/Tim
1	Clean And Sanitize All The Desks And Tables										
2	Clean And Sanitize All The Counter Tops And Surface Areas										
3	Wipe Down The Walls Wherever There Are Spills And Splashes										
4	Disinfect Touch Points, Light Switches And Other Switches										
5	Clean And Disinfect All Doors, Handles And Doorknobs										
6	Clean And Dust Door Frames, Remember To Dust The Tops										
7	Dust Light Fixtures & Shades With A Duster Or A Microfibre Cloth										
8	Clean And Wipe Mirrors Remove Fingerprints, Smears & Dirt										
9	Clean And Sanitize Over Chair Tables										
10	Clean And Polish Bookshelves, Remember To Dust The Top										
11	Remove, Wash And Clean Any Dirty Cups Or Glasses										
12	Remove, Wash And Clean Any Dirty Plates, Bowels Or Cutlery										
13	Clean And Sanitize Any Chairs, Seats And Benches										
14	Water Jugs (Washed Thoroughly Each Day & Re-Filled)										
15	Water Any Plants And Flowers										
16	Dust Plant Leafs (A Healthy Plant Needs To Be Clear Of Dust)										
17	Empty The Waste Baskets And Recycling Bins										
18	Clean And Disinfectant The Waste Bins And Recycling Bins										
19	Clean And Wipe Down Windowsills										
20	Spray Air Freshener This Keeps The Room Smelling Fresh										
21	Clean And Disinfect Cabinets And Units										
22	Clean And Sanitize Desk Accessories										
23	Replace Dirty Table Linen And Move To Laundry Room										
24	Polish Any Wooden Furniture And Hardwood Surfaces										
25	Clean Skirting Boards/Baseboards And Corners										
26	Clean And Polish Fireplace Mantelpiece And Surrounds										
27	Wipe Down Equipment & Sanitize Tea And Coffee Making Facilities										
28	Clean And Sanitize Telephones, Cords/Leads & All Touch Points										
29	Clean And Sanitize Walking Sticks And Any Other Walking Aids										

Care Home Cleaning Tasks - Communal Area	M	T	W	T	F	S	S	Cleaned By	Checked By	Date/Time
Dust Television, Top Sides And Back, TV Unit And TV Stand										
Clean TV Screen With Soft Damp Cloth (Use Water/Cleaner)										
Vacuum/Hoover Between Furniture And The Walls										
Clean And Sanitize All Wheelchairs										
Check For Broken Wheelchairs, Frames and Wheels										
Vacuum Under Furniture, Units, Tables And Cabinets										
Vacuum And Hoover The Carpets, Mats And Rugs										
Vacuum Furnishings, Cushions, Chairs, Sofas And Couches										
Steam Clean Carpets And Rugs										
Dust And Clean Any Picture Frames And Wall Art										
Clean & Check Contents Of Medicine Trolleys & Cupboards										
Clean & Vacuum The Desk Chair, Legs And Chair Wheels										
Wash And Clean Air Vents										
Dust Ceiling Fan Blades With Duster Or A Microfibre Cloth										
Wash And Clean Windows (Inside And Outside)										
Dust And Clean The Walls From Top To Bottom										
Clean Blinds (Dust The Blinds With A Damp Microfibre Cloth)										
Clean Curtains (Vacuum On A Low Setting Or Wash If Possible)										
Dust And Wash Radiator Covers										
Wash And Clean Ceiling Light Covers										
Clean & Vacuum Central Heating Units (Backs Of Radiators)										
Clean And Disinfect Any Handrails										
Clean And Sanitize Computer, Keyboard And Computer Mice										
Clean And Sanitize iPads, Tablets, Laptops & Mobile Phones										
Floors Mopped Clean With Cleaning Or Disinfecting Solution										
The Floors Are Swept And Free From Debris And Litter										
Clean Sliding Doors and Room Partitions										
Throw Away Outdated Newspapers, Magazines, Papers										
Check For Broken Furniture (Report/Schedule Maintenance)										
Light Bulbs Checked And None Functioning Bulbs Replaced										
Check Hardware, Door Stops And Lock Mechanisms										
Fire Exit Lights And Emergency Lights Checked & Functioning										
Test Carbon Monoxide Alarm And Replace Batteries If Required										
Test Smoke Detector Alarm And Replace Batteries If Required										
Paper Dispensers And Paper Towel Rolls Re-Stocked										
Soap Dispensers, Hand Sanitizers And Hand Gels Are Refilled										
Face Masks, Protective Gloves And Face Shields Re-Stocked										

CARE HOME TOILET & RESTROOM CLEANING *Checklist*

Building	Location	Room Number	Area

Start Date & Time	Finnish Date & Time	Name	Signature

	Care Home Cleaning Tasks - Toilet & Restroom	M	T	W	T	F	S	S	Cleaned By	Checked By	Date/Tim
1	Clean And Sanitize All The Counter Tops And Surface Areas										
2	Wipe Down The Walls Wherever There Are Spills And Splashes										
3	Disinfect Touch Points, Light Switches And Other Switches										
4	Clean And Disinfect All Doors, Handles And Doorknobs										
5	Clean And Dust Door Frames, Remember To Dust The Tops										
6	Dust Light Fixtures With A Duster Or A Microfibre Cloth										
7	Wall Mirrors Cleaned With Glass Cleaner										
8	Clean Any Bathroom Glasses And Cups										
9	Clean And Sanitize Any Chairs And Seats										
10	Empty The Waste Basket And Recycling Bin										
11	Clean And Disinfectant The Waste Bin And Recycling Bin										
12	Clean And Wipe Down Windowsills										
13	Spray Air Freshener This Keeps The Room Smelling Fresh										
14	Air/Odour Control Systems Are Filled And Operating Correctly										
15	Clean Skirting Boards/Baseboards And Corners										
16	Vacuum And Hoover Bath Mats, Shower Mats And Rugs										
17	Replace Bath Mats, Shower Mats And Rugs With Clean Ones										
18	Steam Clean Carpets And Rugs										
19	Hand Towels Replaced With Fresh Clean Ones										
20	Bath Towels Replaced With Fresh Clean Ones										
21	Face Towels Replaced With Fresh Clean Ones										
22	Electric Hand Dryers Cleaned, Disinfected & Operating Correctly										
23	Soap Dispensers, Sanitizers And Hand Gels Are Refilled										
24	Clean & Check Contents Of Medicine Trolleys & Cupboards										
25	Clean And Disinfect Any Handrails										
26	Sinks, Taps And Fixtures Cleaned And Disinfected										
27	Clean And Disinfect Cabinets And Units										
28	Feminine Hygiene Dispensers Re-Stocked										
29	Feminine Hygiene Bins/Containers Emptied And Cleared										

Care Home Cleaning Tasks - Toilet & Restroom	M	T	W	T	F	S	S	Cleaned By	Checked By	Date/Time
Clean & Vacuum Central Heating Units (Backs Of Radiators)										
Wash And Clean Ceiling Light Covers										
Toilet Roll Holders And Toilet Rolls Re-Stocked										
Toilet Roll Holders Cleaned And Disinfected										
Clean Inside The Toilets And Urinals With Disinfectant										
Toilet Seats Cleaned And Disinfected										
Clean Top Of Toilets Tanks, The Bases And Behind Toilets										
Urinal Handles Cleaned And Disinfected										
Urinal Screens Cleaned, Disinfected And Blocks Replaced										
Paper Dispensers And Paper Towel Rolls Re-Stocked										
Paper Dispensers And Paper Towel Roll Cleaned & Disinfected										
The Floors Are Swept And Free From Debris And Litter										
Floors Mopped Clean With Cleaning Or Disinfecting Solution										
Put Up Or Place Wet Floor Signs After Mopping Floors										
Showers And Shower Heads, Cleaned And Disinfected										
Soak Shower Heads										
Clean And Disinfect Glass Shower Doors/Outer Doors										
Clean Soap Scum From Shower Walls										
Clean Blinds (Dust The Blinds With A Damp Microfibre Cloth)										
Clean Curtains (Vacuum On A Low Setting Or Wash If Possible)										
Dust And Wash Radiator Covers										
Clean And Disinfect Commodes Between Each Use										
Clean And Disinfect Shower Chairs Between Each Use										
Bath Hoists Cleaned And Disinfected Between Each Use										
Scrub Tub/Bath, Polish Facets And Taps, Clean & Disinfected										
Toothbrush Holders And Soap Holders Cleaned										
Re-Place Shower Curtains With Clean Fresh Ones										
Wash And Clean Air Vents										
Thoroughly Clean Grout And Tiles										
Disinfect And Clean All The Walls From Top To Bottom										
Wash And Clean Windows (Inside And Outside)										
Unclog The Drains (Sink, Bath And Shower)										
Pour Drain Cleaner Down Sink, Shower & Bath Drains										
Floor Drains And Drain Covers Are Open And Free Of Debris										
Hair Dryers Cleaned And Disinfected And Operating Correctly										
Light Bulbs Checked And None Functioning Bulbs Replaced										
Check Hardware, Door Stops And Lock Mechanisms										

CARE HOME BEDROOM CLEANING *Checklist*

Building	Location	Room Number	Area

Start Date & Time	Finnish Date & Time	Name	Signature

	Care Home Cleaning Tasks - Bedrooms	M	T	W	T	F	S	S	Cleaned By	Checked By	Date/Tim
1	Clean And Sanitize All The Desks And Tables										
2	Clean And Sanitize All The Counter Tops And Surface Areas										
3	Wipe Down The Walls Wherever There Are Spills And Splashes										
4	Disinfect Touch Points, Light Switches And Other Switches										
5	Clean And Disinfect All Doors, Handles And Doorknobs										
6	Clean And Dust Door Frames, Remember To Dust The Tops										
7	Dust Light Fixtures With A Duster Or A Microfibre Cloth										
8	Clean & Wipe Mirrors Remove Fingerprints, Smears & Dirt										
9	Clean And Dust Bedside Cabinets										
10	Clean And Sanitize Over Chair Tables										
11	Clean And Sanitize Over Bed Tables										
12	Clean And Check Bed Frames										
13	Mattresses Hoovered And Cleaned With Disinfectant										
14	Clean And Polish Bookshelves, Remember To Dust The Top										
15	Remove, Wash And Clean Any Dirty Cups Or Glasses										
16	Remove, Wash And Clean Any Dirty Plates, Bowels Or Cutlery										
17	Clean And Sanitize Any Chairs And Seats										
18	Water Jug (Washed Thoroughly Each Day & Re-Filled)										
19	Water Any Plants And Flowers										
20	Dust Plant Leafs (A Healthy Plant Needs To Be Clear Of Dust)										
21	Empty The Waste Basket And Recycling Bin										
22	Clean And Disinfectant The Waste Bin And Recycling Bin										
23	Clean And Wipe Down Windowsills										
24	Spray Air Freshener This Keeps The Room Smelling Fresh										
25	Clean And Disinfect Cabinets And Units										
26	Clean And Sanitize Desk Accessories										
27	Replace Dirty Linen And Move To Laundry Room										
28	Polish Any Wooden Furniture And Hardwood Surfaces										
29	Clean Skirting Boards/Baseboards And Corners										

Care Home Cleaning Tasks - Bedrooms Continued	M	T	W	T	F	S	S	Cleaned By	Checked By	Date/Time
Dust Television, Top Sides And Back, TV Unit And TV Stand										
Clean TV Screen With Soft Damp Cloth (Use Water/Cleaner)										
Vacuum/Hoover Between Bedroom Furniture And The Walls										
Clean And Sanitize Resident's Personal Wheelchair										
Check For Broken Wheelchairs, Frames and Wheels										
Vacuum Under Furniture, Beds, Sofas and Dressers										
Vacuum And Hoover The Carpets, Mats And Rugs										
Vacuum Furnishings, Cushions, Chairs, Sofas And Couches										
Steam Clean Carpets And Rugs										
Dust And Clean Any Picture Frames And Photo Frames										
Ledges, Flat Surfaces And The Tops Of Wardrobes Dusted										
Clean & Check Contents Of Medicine Trolleys & Cupboards										
Clean And Sanitize Mobile Phone, Phone Case And Screen										
Clean & Vacuum The Desk Chair, Legs And Chair Wheels										
Wash And Clean Air Vents										
Dust Ceiling Fan Blades With Duster Or A Microfibre Cloth										
Wash And Clean Windows (Inside And Outside)										
Dust And Clean The Walls From Top To Bottom										
Clean Blinds (Dust The Blinds With A Damp Microfibre Cloth)										
Clean Curtains (Vacuum On A Low Setting Or Wash If Possible)										
Dust And Wash Radiator Covers										
Wash And Clean Ceiling Light Covers										
Clean & Vacuum Central Heating Units (Backs Of Radiators)										
Clean And Disinfect Any Handrails										
Hand Towels Replaced With Fresh Clean Ones										
Sink Wall Mirror Cleaned With Glass Cleaner										
Sinks, Taps And Fixtures Cleaned And Disinfected										
Pour Drain Cleaner Down Sink Drains										
Check For Broken Furniture (Report/Schedule Maintenance)										
Light Bulbs Checked And None Functioning Bulbs Replaced										
Check Hardware, Door Stops And Lock Mechanisms										
Fire Exit Lights And Emergency Lights Checked & Functioning										
Test Carbon Monoxide Alarm And Replace Batteries If Required										
Test Smoke Detector Alarm And Replace Batteries If Required										
Paper Dispensers And Paper Towel Rolls Re-Stocked										
Soap Dispensers, Hand Sanitizers And Hand Gels Are Refilled										
Face Masks, Protective Gloves And Face Shields Re-Stocked										

CARE HOME COMMUNAL AREA CLEANING *Checklist*

Building	Location	Room Number	Area

Start Date & Time	Finnish Date & Time	Name	Signature

	Care Home Cleaning Tasks - Communal Area	M	T	W	T	F	S	S	Cleaned By	Checked By	Date/Tim
1	Clean And Sanitize All The Desks And Tables										
2	Clean And Sanitize All The Counter Tops And Surface Areas										
3	Wipe Down The Walls Wherever There Are Spills And Splashes										
4	Disinfect Touch Points, Light Switches And Other Switches										
5	Clean And Disinfect All Doors, Handles And Doorknobs										
6	Clean And Dust Door Frames, Remember To Dust The Tops										
7	Dust Light Fixtures & Shades With A Duster Or A Microfibre Cloth										
8	Clean And Wipe Mirrors Remove Fingerprints, Smears & Dirt										
9	Clean And Sanitize Over Chair Tables										
10	Clean And Polish Bookshelves, Remember To Dust The Top										
11	Remove, Wash And Clean Any Dirty Cups Or Glasses										
12	Remove, Wash And Clean Any Dirty Plates, Bowels Or Cutlery										
13	Clean And Sanitize Any Chairs, Seats And Benches										
14	Water Jugs (Washed Thoroughly Each Day & Re-Filled)										
15	Water Any Plants And Flowers										
16	Dust Plant Leafs (A Healthy Plant Needs To Be Clear Of Dust)										
17	Empty The Waste Baskets And Recycling Bins										
18	Clean And Disinfectant The Waste Bins And Recycling Bins										
19	Clean And Wipe Down Windowsills										
20	Spray Air Freshener This Keeps The Room Smelling Fresh										
21	Clean And Disinfect Cabinets And Units										
22	Clean And Sanitize Desk Accessories										
23	Replace Dirty Table Linen And Move To Laundry Room										
24	Polish Any Wooden Furniture And Hardwood Surfaces										
25	Clean Skirting Boards/Baseboards And Corners										
26	Clean And Polish Fireplace Mantelpiece And Surrounds										
27	Wipe Down Equipment & Sanitize Tea And Coffee Making Facilities										
28	Clean And Sanitize Telephones, Cords/Leads & All Touch Points										
29	Clean And Sanitize Walking Sticks And Any Other Walking Aids										

Care Home Cleaning Tasks - Communal Area	M	T	W	T	F	S	S	Cleaned By	Checked By	Date/Time
Dust Television, Top Sides And Back, TV Unit And TV Stand										
Clean TV Screen With Soft Damp Cloth (Use Water/Cleaner)										
Vacuum/Hoover Between Furniture And The Walls										
Clean And Sanitize All Wheelchairs										
Check For Broken Wheelchairs, Frames and Wheels										
Vacuum Under Furniture, Units, Tables And Cabinets										
Vacuum And Hoover The Carpets, Mats And Rugs										
Vacuum Furnishings, Cushions, Chairs, Sofas And Couches										
Steam Clean Carpets And Rugs										
Dust And Clean Any Picture Frames And Wall Art										
Clean & Check Contents Of Medicine Trolleys & Cupboards										
Clean & Vacuum The Desk Chair, Legs And Chair Wheels										
Wash And Clean Air Vents										
Dust Ceiling Fan Blades With Duster Or A Microfibre Cloth										
Wash And Clean Windows (Inside And Outside)										
Dust And Clean The Walls From Top To Bottom										
Clean Blinds (Dust The Blinds With A Damp Microfibre Cloth)										
Clean Curtains (Vacuum On A Low Setting Or Wash If Possible)										
Dust And Wash Radiator Covers										
Wash And Clean Ceiling Light Covers										
Clean & Vacuum Central Heating Units (Backs Of Radiators)										
Clean And Disinfect Any Handrails										
Clean And Sanitize Computer, Keyboard And Computer Mice										
Clean And Sanitize iPads, Tablets, Laptops & Mobile Phones										
Floors Mopped Clean With Cleaning Or Disinfecting Solution										
The Floors Are Swept And Free From Debris And Litter										
Clean Sliding Doors and Room Partitions										
Throw Away Outdated Newspapers, Magazines, Papers										
Check For Broken Furniture (Report/Schedule Maintenance)										
Light Bulbs Checked And None Functioning Bulbs Replaced										
Check Hardware, Door Stops And Lock Mechanisms										
Fire Exit Lights And Emergency Lights Checked & Functioning										
Test Carbon Monoxide Alarm And Replace Batteries If Required										
Test Smoke Detector Alarm And Replace Batteries If Required										
Paper Dispensers And Paper Towel Rolls Re-Stocked										
Soap Dispensers, Hand Sanitizers And Hand Gels Are Refilled										
Face Masks, Protective Gloves And Face Shields Re-Stocked										

CARE HOME TOILET & RESTROOM CLEANING *Checklist*

Building	Location	Room Number	Area

Start Date & Time	Finnish Date & Time	Name	Signature

	Care Home Cleaning Tasks - Toilet & Restroom	M	T	W	T	F	S	S	Cleaned By	Checked By	Date/Time
1	Clean And Sanitize All The Counter Tops And Surface Areas										
2	Wipe Down The Walls Wherever There Are Spills And Splashes										
3	Disinfect Touch Points, Light Switches And Other Switches										
4	Clean And Disinfect All Doors, Handles And Doorknobs										
5	Clean And Dust Door Frames, Remember To Dust The Tops										
6	Dust Light Fixtures With A Duster Or A Microfibre Cloth										
7	Wall Mirrors Cleaned With Glass Cleaner										
8	Clean Any Bathroom Glasses And Cups										
9	Clean And Sanitize Any Chairs And Seats										
10	Empty The Waste Basket And Recycling Bin										
11	Clean And Disinfectant The Waste Bin And Recycling Bin										
12	Clean And Wipe Down Windowsills										
13	Spray Air Freshener This Keeps The Room Smelling Fresh										
14	Air/Odour Control Systems Are Filled And Operating Correctly										
15	Clean Skirting Boards/Baseboards And Corners										
16	Vacuum And Hoover Bath Mats, Shower Mats And Rugs										
17	Replace Bath Mats, Shower Mats And Rugs With Clean Ones										
18	Steam Clean Carpets And Rugs										
19	Hand Towels Replaced With Fresh Clean Ones										
20	Bath Towels Replaced With Fresh Clean Ones										
21	Face Towels Replaced With Fresh Clean Ones										
22	Electric Hand Dryers Cleaned, Disinfected & Operating Correctly										
23	Soap Dispensers, Sanitizers And Hand Gels Are Refilled										
24	Clean & Check Contents Of Medicine Trolleys & Cupboards										
25	Clean And Disinfect Any Handrails										
26	Sinks, Taps And Fixtures Cleaned And Disinfected										
27	Clean And Disinfect Cabinets And Units										
28	Feminine Hygiene Dispensers Re-Stocked										
29	Feminine Hygiene Bins/Containers Emptied And Cleared										

Care Home Cleaning Tasks - Toilet & Restroom	M	T	W	T	F	S	S	Cleaned By	Checked By	Date/Time
Clean & Vacuum Central Heating Units (Backs Of Radiators)										
Wash And Clean Ceiling Light Covers										
Toilet Roll Holders And Toilet Rolls Re-Stocked										
Toilet Roll Holders Cleaned And Disinfected										
Clean Inside The Toilets And Urinals With Disinfectant										
Toilet Seats Cleaned And Disinfected										
Clean Top Of Toilets Tanks, The Bases And Behind Toilets										
Urinal Handles Cleaned And Disinfected										
Urinal Screens Cleaned, Disinfected And Blocks Replaced										
Paper Dispensers And Paper Towel Rolls Re-Stocked										
Paper Dispensers And Paper Towel Roll Cleaned & Disinfected										
The Floors Are Swept And Free From Debris And Litter										
Floors Mopped Clean With Cleaning Or Disinfecting Solution										
Put Up Or Place Wet Floor Signs After Mopping Floors										
Showers And Shower Heads, Cleaned And Disinfected										
Soak Shower Heads										
Clean And Disinfect Glass Shower Doors/Outer Doors										
Clean Soap Scum From Shower Walls										
Clean Blinds (Dust The Blinds With A Damp Microfibre Cloth)										
Clean Curtains (Vacuum On A Low Setting Or Wash If Possible)										
Dust And Wash Radiator Covers										
Clean And Disinfect Commodes Between Each Use										
Clean And Disinfect Shower Chairs Between Each Use										
Bath Hoists Cleaned And Disinfected Between Each Use										
Scrub Tub/Bath, Polish Facets And Taps, Clean & Disinfected										
Toothbrush Holders And Soap Holders Cleaned										
Re-Place Shower Curtains With Clean Fresh Ones										
Wash And Clean Air Vents										
Thoroughly Clean Grout And Tiles										
Disinfect And Clean All The Walls From Top To Bottom										
Wash And Clean Windows (Inside And Outside)										
Unclog The Drains (Sink, Bath And Shower)										
Pour Drain Cleaner Down Sink, Shower & Bath Drains										
Floor Drains And Drain Covers Are Open And Free Of Debris										
Hair Dryers Cleaned And Disinfected And Operating Correctly										
Light Bulbs Checked And None Functioning Bulbs Replaced										
Check Hardware, Door Stops And Lock Mechanisms										

CARE HOME BEDROOM CLEANING *Checklist*

Building	Location	Room Number	Area

Start Date & Time	Finnish Date & Time	Name	Signature

	Care Home Cleaning Tasks - Bedrooms	M	T	W	T	F	S	S	Cleaned By	Checked By	Date/Ti
1	Clean And Sanitize All The Desks And Tables										
2	Clean And Sanitize All The Counter Tops And Surface Areas										
3	Wipe Down The Walls Wherever There Are Spills And Splashes										
4	Disinfect Touch Points, Light Switches And Other Switches										
5	Clean And Disinfect All Doors, Handles And Doorknobs										
6	Clean And Dust Door Frames, Remember To Dust The Tops										
7	Dust Light Fixtures With A Duster Or A Microfibre Cloth										
8	Clean & Wipe Mirrors Remove Fingerprints, Smears & Dirt										
9	Clean And Dust Bedside Cabinets										
10	Clean And Sanitize Over Chair Tables										
11	Clean And Sanitize Over Bed Tables										
12	Clean And Check Bed Frames										
13	Mattresses Hoovered And Cleaned With Disinfectant										
14	Clean And Polish Bookshelves, Remember To Dust The Top										
15	Remove, Wash And Clean Any Dirty Cups Or Glasses										
16	Remove, Wash And Clean Any Dirty Plates, Bowels Or Cutlery										
17	Clean And Sanitize Any Chairs And Seats										
18	Water Jug (Washed Thoroughly Each Day & Re-Filled)										
19	Water Any Plants And Flowers										
20	Dust Plant Leafs (A Healthy Plant Needs To Be Clear Of Dust)										
21	Empty The Waste Basket And Recycling Bin										
22	Clean And Disinfectant The Waste Bin And Recycling Bin										
23	Clean And Wipe Down Windowsills										
24	Spray Air Freshener This Keeps The Room Smelling Fresh										
25	Clean And Disinfect Cabinets And Units										
26	Clean And Sanitize Desk Accessories										
27	Replace Dirty Linen And Move To Laundry Room										
28	Polish Any Wooden Furniture And Hardwood Surfaces										
29	Clean Skirting Boards/Baseboards And Corners										

Care Home Cleaning Tasks - Bedrooms Continued	M	T	W	T	F	S	S	Cleaned By	Checked By	Date/Time
Dust Television, Top Sides And Back, TV Unit And TV Stand										
Clean TV Screen With Soft Damp Cloth (Use Water/Cleaner)										
Vacuum/Hoover Between Bedroom Furniture And The Walls										
Clean And Sanitize Resident's Personal Wheelchair										
Check For Broken Wheelchairs, Frames and Wheels										
Vacuum Under Furniture, Beds, Sofas and Dressers										
Vacuum And Hoover The Carpets, Mats And Rugs										
Vacuum Furnishings, Cushions, Chairs, Sofas And Couches										
Steam Clean Carpets And Rugs										
Dust And Clean Any Picture Frames And Photo Frames										
Ledges, Flat Surfaces And The Tops Of Wardrobes Dusted										
Clean & Check Contents Of Medicine Trolleys & Cupboards										
Clean And Sanitize Mobile Phone, Phone Case And Screen										
Clean & Vacuum The Desk Chair, Legs And Chair Wheels										
Wash And Clean Air Vents										
Dust Ceiling Fan Blades With Duster Or A Microfibre Cloth										
Wash And Clean Windows (Inside And Outside)										
Dust And Clean The Walls From Top To Bottom										
Clean Blinds (Dust The Blinds With A Damp Microfibre Cloth)										
Clean Curtains (Vacuum On A Low Setting Or Wash If Possible)										
Dust And Wash Radiator Covers										
Wash And Clean Ceiling Light Covers										
Clean & Vacuum Central Heating Units (Backs Of Radiators)										
Clean And Disinfect Any Handrails										
Hand Towels Replaced With Fresh Clean Ones										
Sink Wall Mirror Cleaned With Glass Cleaner										
Sinks, Taps And Fixtures Cleaned And Disinfected										
Pour Drain Cleaner Down Sink Drains										
Check For Broken Furniture (Report/Schedule Maintenance)										
Light Bulbs Checked And None Functioning Bulbs Replaced										
Check Hardware, Door Stops And Lock Mechanisms										
Fire Exit Lights And Emergency Lights Checked & Functioning										
Test Carbon Monoxide Alarm And Replace Batteries If Required										
Test Smoke Detector Alarm And Replace Batteries If Required										
Paper Dispensers And Paper Towel Rolls Re-Stocked										
Soap Dispensers, Hand Sanitizers And Hand Gels Are Refilled										
Face Masks, Protective Gloves And Face Shields Re-Stocked										

CARE HOME COMMUNAL AREA CLEANING *Checklist*

Building	Location	Room Number	Area

Start Date & Time	Finnish Date & Time	Name	Signature

	Care Home Cleaning Tasks - Communal Area	M	T	W	T	F	S	S	Cleaned By	Checked By	Date/Tim
1	Clean And Sanitize All The Desks And Tables										
2	Clean And Sanitize All The Counter Tops And Surface Areas										
3	Wipe Down The Walls Wherever There Are Spills And Splashes										
4	Disinfect Touch Points, Light Switches And Other Switches										
5	Clean And Disinfect All Doors, Handles And Doorknobs										
6	Clean And Dust Door Frames, Remember To Dust The Tops										
7	Dust Light Fixtures & Shades With A Duster Or A Microfibre Cloth										
8	Clean And Wipe Mirrors Remove Fingerprints, Smears & Dirt										
9	Clean And Sanitize Over Chair Tables										
10	Clean And Polish Bookshelves, Remember To Dust The Top										
11	Remove, Wash And Clean Any Dirty Cups Or Glasses										
12	Remove, Wash And Clean Any Dirty Plates, Bowels Or Cutlery										
13	Clean And Sanitize Any Chairs, Seats And Benches										
14	Water Jugs (Washed Thoroughly Each Day & Re-Filled)										
15	Water Any Plants And Flowers										
16	Dust Plant Leafs (A Healthy Plant Needs To Be Clear Of Dust)										
17	Empty The Waste Baskets And Recycling Bins										
18	Clean And Disinfectant The Waste Bins And Recycling Bins										
19	Clean And Wipe Down Windowsills										
20	Spray Air Freshener This Keeps The Room Smelling Fresh										
21	Clean And Disinfect Cabinets And Units										
22	Clean And Sanitize Desk Accessories										
23	Replace Dirty Table Linen And Move To Laundry Room										
24	Polish Any Wooden Furniture And Hardwood Surfaces										
25	Clean Skirting Boards/Baseboards And Corners										
26	Clean And Polish Fireplace Mantelpiece And Surrounds										
27	Wipe Down Equipment & Sanitize Tea And Coffee Making Facilities										
28	Clean And Sanitize Telephones, Cords/Leads & All Touch Points										
29	Clean And Sanitize Walking Sticks And Any Other Walking Aids										

Care Home Cleaning Tasks - Communal Area	M	T	W	T	F	S	S	Cleaned By	Checked By	Date/Time
Dust Television, Top Sides And Back, TV Unit And TV Stand										
Clean TV Screen With Soft Damp Cloth (Use Water/Cleaner)										
Vacuum/Hoover Between Furniture And The Walls										
Clean And Sanitize All Wheelchairs										
Check For Broken Wheelchairs, Frames and Wheels										
Vacuum Under Furniture, Units, Tables And Cabinets										
Vacuum And Hoover The Carpets, Mats And Rugs										
Vacuum Furnishings, Cushions, Chairs, Sofas And Couches										
Steam Clean Carpets And Rugs										
Dust And Clean Any Picture Frames And Wall Art										
Clean & Check Contents Of Medicine Trolleys & Cupboards										
Clean & Vacuum The Desk Chair, Legs And Chair Wheels										
Wash And Clean Air Vents										
Dust Ceiling Fan Blades With Duster Or A Microfibre Cloth										
Wash And Clean Windows (Inside And Outside)										
Dust And Clean The Walls From Top To Bottom										
Clean Blinds (Dust The Blinds With A Damp Microfibre Cloth)										
Clean Curtains (Vacuum On A Low Setting Or Wash If Possible)										
Dust And Wash Radiator Covers										
Wash And Clean Ceiling Light Covers										
Clean & Vacuum Central Heating Units (Backs Of Radiators)										
Clean And Disinfect Any Handrails										
Clean And Sanitize Computer, Keyboard And Computer Mice										
Clean And Sanitize iPads, Tablets, Laptops & Mobile Phones										
Floors Mopped Clean With Cleaning Or Disinfecting Solution										
The Floors Are Swept And Free From Debris And Litter										
Clean Sliding Doors and Room Partitions										
Throw Away Outdated Newspapers, Magazines, Papers										
Check For Broken Furniture (Report/Schedule Maintenance)										
Light Bulbs Checked And None Functioning Bulbs Replaced										
Check Hardware, Door Stops And Lock Mechanisms										
Fire Exit Lights And Emergency Lights Checked & Functioning										
Test Carbon Monoxide Alarm And Replace Batteries If Required										
Test Smoke Detector Alarm And Replace Batteries If Required										
Paper Dispensers And Paper Towel Rolls Re-Stocked										
Soap Dispensers, Hand Sanitizers And Hand Gels Are Refilled										
Face Masks, Protective Gloves And Face Shields Re-Stocked										

CARE HOME TOILET & RESTROOM CLEANING *Checklist*

Building	Location	Room Number	Area

Start Date & Time	Finnish Date & Time	Name	Signature

	Care Home Cleaning Tasks - Toilet & Restroom	M	T	W	T	F	S	S	Cleaned By	Checked By	Date/Tin
1	Clean And Sanitize All The Counter Tops And Surface Areas										
2	Wipe Down The Walls Wherever There Are Spills And Splashes										
3	Disinfect Touch Points, Light Switches And Other Switches										
4	Clean And Disinfect All Doors, Handles And Doorknobs										
5	Clean And Dust Door Frames, Remember To Dust The Tops										
6	Dust Light Fixtures With A Duster Or A Microfibre Cloth										
7	Wall Mirrors Cleaned With Glass Cleaner										
8	Clean Any Bathroom Glasses And Cups										
9	Clean And Sanitize Any Chairs And Seats										
10	Empty The Waste Basket And Recycling Bin										
11	Clean And Disinfectant The Waste Bin And Recycling Bin										
12	Clean And Wipe Down Windowsills										
13	Spray Air Freshener This Keeps The Room Smelling Fresh										
14	Air/Odour Control Systems Are Filled And Operating Correctly										
15	Clean Skirting Boards/Baseboards And Corners										
16	Vacuum And Hoover Bath Mats, Shower Mats And Rugs										
17	Replace Bath Mats, Shower Mats And Rugs With Clean Ones										
18	Steam Clean Carpets And Rugs										
19	Hand Towels Replaced With Fresh Clean Ones										
20	Bath Towels Replaced With Fresh Clean Ones										
21	Face Towels Replaced With Fresh Clean Ones										
22	Electric Hand Dryers Cleaned, Disinfected & Operating Correctly										
23	Soap Dispensers, Sanitizers And Hand Gels Are Refilled										
24	Clean & Check Contents Of Medicine Trolleys & Cupboards										
25	Clean And Disinfect Any Handrails										
26	Sinks, Taps And Fixtures Cleaned And Disinfected										
27	Clean And Disinfect Cabinets And Units										
28	Feminine Hygiene Dispensers Re-Stocked										
29	Feminine Hygiene Bins/Containers Emptied And Cleared										

Care Home Cleaning Tasks - Toilet & Restroom	M	T	W	T	F	S	S	Cleaned By	Checked By	Date/Time
Clean & Vacuum Central Heating Units (Backs Of Radiators)										
Wash And Clean Ceiling Light Covers										
Toilet Roll Holders And Toilet Rolls Re-Stocked										
Toilet Roll Holders Cleaned And Disinfected										
Clean Inside The Toilets And Urinals With Disinfectant										
Toilet Seats Cleaned And Disinfected										
Clean Top Of Toilets Tanks, The Bases And Behind Toilets										
Urinal Handles Cleaned And Disinfected										
Urinal Screens Cleaned, Disinfected And Blocks Replaced										
Paper Dispensers And Paper Towel Rolls Re-Stocked										
Paper Dispensers And Paper Towel Roll Cleaned & Disinfected										
The Floors Are Swept And Free From Debris And Litter										
Floors Mopped Clean With Cleaning Or Disinfecting Solution										
Put Up Or Place Wet Floor Signs After Mopping Floors										
Showers And Shower Heads, Cleaned And Disinfected										
Soak Shower Heads										
Clean And Disinfect Glass Shower Doors/Outer Doors										
Clean Soap Scum From Shower Walls										
Clean Blinds (Dust The Blinds With A Damp Microfibre Cloth)										
Clean Curtains (Vacuum On A Low Setting Or Wash If Possible)										
Dust And Wash Radiator Covers										
Clean And Disinfect Commodes Between Each Use										
Clean And Disinfect Shower Chairs Between Each Use										
Bath Hoists Cleaned And Disinfected Between Each Use										
Scrub Tub/Bath, Polish Facets And Taps, Clean & Disinfected										
Toothbrush Holders And Soap Holders Cleaned										
Re-Place Shower Curtains With Clean Fresh Ones										
Wash And Clean Air Vents										
Thoroughly Clean Grout And Tiles										
Disinfect And Clean All The Walls From Top To Bottom										
Wash And Clean Windows (Inside And Outside)										
Unclog The Drains (Sink, Bath And Shower)										
Pour Drain Cleaner Down Sink, Shower & Bath Drains										
Floor Drains And Drain Covers Are Open And Free Of Debris										
Hair Dryers Cleaned And Disinfected And Operating Correctly										
Light Bulbs Checked And None Functioning Bulbs Replaced										
Check Hardware, Door Stops And Lock Mechanisms										

CARE HOME BEDROOM CLEANING *Checklist*

Building	Location	Room Number	Area

Start Date & Time	Finnish Date & Time	Name	Signature

	Care Home Cleaning Tasks - Bedrooms	M	T	W	T	F	S	S	Cleaned By	Checked By	Date/Tim
1	Clean And Sanitize All The Desks And Tables										
2	Clean And Sanitize All The Counter Tops And Surface Areas										
3	Wipe Down The Walls Wherever There Are Spills And Splashes										
4	Disinfect Touch Points, Light Switches And Other Switches										
5	Clean And Disinfect All Doors, Handles And Doorknobs										
6	Clean And Dust Door Frames, Remember To Dust The Tops										
7	Dust Light Fixtures With A Duster Or A Microfibre Cloth										
8	Clean & Wipe Mirrors Remove Fingerprints, Smears & Dirt										
9	Clean And Dust Bedside Cabinets										
10	Clean And Sanitize Over Chair Tables										
11	Clean And Sanitize Over Bed Tables										
12	Clean And Check Bed Frames										
13	Mattresses Hoovered And Cleaned With Disinfectant										
14	Clean And Polish Bookshelves, Remember To Dust The Top										
15	Remove, Wash And Clean Any Dirty Cups Or Glasses										
16	Remove, Wash And Clean Any Dirty Plates, Bowels Or Cutlery										
17	Clean And Sanitize Any Chairs And Seats										
18	Water Jug (Washed Thoroughly Each Day & Re-Filled)										
19	Water Any Plants And Flowers										
20	Dust Plant Leafs (A Healthy Plant Needs To Be Clear Of Dust)										
21	Empty The Waste Basket And Recycling Bin										
22	Clean And Disinfectant The Waste Bin And Recycling Bin										
23	Clean And Wipe Down Windowsills										
24	Spray Air Freshener This Keeps The Room Smelling Fresh										
25	Clean And Disinfect Cabinets And Units										
26	Clean And Sanitize Desk Accessories										
27	Replace Dirty Linen And Move To Laundry Room										
28	Polish Any Wooden Furniture And Hardwood Surfaces										
29	Clean Skirting Boards/Baseboards And Corners										

Care Home Cleaning Tasks - Bedrooms Continued	M	T	W	T	F	S	S	Cleaned By	Checked By	Date/Time
Dust Television, Top Sides And Back, TV Unit And TV Stand										
Clean TV Screen With Soft Damp Cloth (Use Water/Cleaner)										
Vacuum/Hoover Between Bedroom Furniture And The Walls										
Clean And Sanitize Resident's Personal Wheelchair										
Check For Broken Wheelchairs, Frames and Wheels										
Vacuum Under Furniture, Beds, Sofas and Dressers										
Vacuum And Hoover The Carpets, Mats And Rugs										
Vacuum Furnishings, Cushions, Chairs, Sofas And Couches										
Steam Clean Carpets And Rugs										
Dust And Clean Any Picture Frames And Photo Frames										
Ledges, Flat Surfaces And The Tops Of Wardrobes Dusted										
Clean & Check Contents Of Medicine Trolleys & Cupboards										
Clean And Sanitize Mobile Phone, Phone Case And Screen										
Clean & Vacuum The Desk Chair, Legs And Chair Wheels										
Wash And Clean Air Vents										
Dust Ceiling Fan Blades With Duster Or A Microfibre Cloth										
Wash And Clean Windows (Inside And Outside)										
Dust And Clean The Walls From Top To Bottom										
Clean Blinds (Dust The Blinds With A Damp Microfibre Cloth)										
Clean Curtains (Vacuum On A Low Setting Or Wash If Possible)										
Dust And Wash Radiator Covers										
Wash And Clean Ceiling Light Covers										
Clean & Vacuum Central Heating Units (Backs Of Radiators)										
Clean And Disinfect Any Handrails										
Hand Towels Replaced With Fresh Clean Ones										
Sink Wall Mirror Cleaned With Glass Cleaner										
Sinks, Taps And Fixtures Cleaned And Disinfected										
Pour Drain Cleaner Down Sink Drains										
Check For Broken Furniture (Report/Schedule Maintenance)										
Light Bulbs Checked And None Functioning Bulbs Replaced										
Check Hardware, Door Stops And Lock Mechanisms										
Fire Exit Lights And Emergency Lights Checked & Functioning										
Test Carbon Monoxide Alarm And Replace Batteries If Required										
Test Smoke Detector Alarm And Replace Batteries If Required										
Paper Dispensers And Paper Towel Rolls Re-Stocked										
Soap Dispensers, Hand Sanitizers And Hand Gels Are Refilled										
Face Masks, Protective Gloves And Face Shields Re-Stocked										

CARE HOME COMMUNAL AREA CLEANING *Checklist*

Building	Location	Room Number	Area

Start Date & Time	Finnish Date & Time	Name	Signature

	Care Home Cleaning Tasks - Communal Area	M	T	W	T	F	S	S	Cleaned By	Checked By	Date/Tin
1	Clean And Sanitize All The Desks And Tables										
2	Clean And Sanitize All The Counter Tops And Surface Areas										
3	Wipe Down The Walls Wherever There Are Spills And Splashes										
4	Disinfect Touch Points, Light Switches And Other Switches										
5	Clean And Disinfect All Doors, Handles And Doorknobs										
6	Clean And Dust Door Frames, Remember To Dust The Tops										
7	Dust Light Fixtures & Shades With A Duster Or A Microfibre Cloth										
8	Clean And Wipe Mirrors Remove Fingerprints, Smears & Dirt										
9	Clean And Sanitize Over Chair Tables										
10	Clean And Polish Bookshelves, Remember To Dust The Top										
11	Remove, Wash And Clean Any Dirty Cups Or Glasses										
12	Remove, Wash And Clean Any Dirty Plates, Bowels Or Cutlery										
13	Clean And Sanitize Any Chairs, Seats And Benches										
14	Water Jugs (Washed Thoroughly Each Day & Re-Filled)										
15	Water Any Plants And Flowers										
16	Dust Plant Leafs (A Healthy Plant Needs To Be Clear Of Dust)										
17	Empty The Waste Baskets And Recycling Bins										
18	Clean And Disinfectant The Waste Bins And Recycling Bins										
19	Clean And Wipe Down Windowsills										
20	Spray Air Freshener This Keeps The Room Smelling Fresh										
21	Clean And Disinfect Cabinets And Units										
22	Clean And Sanitize Desk Accessories										
23	Replace Dirty Table Linen And Move To Laundry Room										
24	Polish Any Wooden Furniture And Hardwood Surfaces										
25	Clean Skirting Boards/Baseboards And Corners										
26	Clean And Polish Fireplace Mantelpiece And Surrounds										
27	Wipe Down Equipment & Sanitize Tea And Coffee Making Facilities										
28	Clean And Sanitize Telephones, Cords/Leads & All Touch Points										
29	Clean And Sanitize Walking Sticks And Any Other Walking Aids										

Care Home Cleaning Tasks - Communal Area	M	T	W	T	F	S	S	Cleaned By	Checked By	Date/Time
Dust Television, Top Sides And Back, TV Unit And TV Stand										
Clean TV Screen With Soft Damp Cloth (Use Water/Cleaner)										
Vacuum/Hoover Between Furniture And The Walls										
Clean And Sanitize All Wheelchairs										
Check For Broken Wheelchairs, Frames and Wheels										
Vacuum Under Furniture, Units, Tables And Cabinets										
Vacuum And Hoover The Carpets, Mats And Rugs										
Vacuum Furnishings, Cushions, Chairs, Sofas And Couches										
Steam Clean Carpets And Rugs										
Dust And Clean Any Picture Frames And Wall Art										
Clean & Check Contents Of Medicine Trolleys & Cupboards										
Clean & Vacuum The Desk Chair, Legs And Chair Wheels										
Wash And Clean Air Vents										
Dust Ceiling Fan Blades With Duster Or A Microfibre Cloth										
Wash And Clean Windows (Inside And Outside)										
Dust And Clean The Walls From Top To Bottom										
Clean Blinds (Dust The Blinds With A Damp Microfibre Cloth)										
Clean Curtains (Vacuum On A Low Setting Or Wash If Possible)										
Dust And Wash Radiator Covers										
Wash And Clean Ceiling Light Covers										
Clean & Vacuum Central Heating Units (Backs Of Radiators)										
Clean And Disinfect Any Handrails										
Clean And Sanitize Computer, Keyboard And Computer Mice										
Clean And Sanitize iPads, Tablets, Laptops & Mobile Phones										
Floors Mopped Clean With Cleaning Or Disinfecting Solution										
The Floors Are Swept And Free From Debris And Litter										
Clean Sliding Doors and Room Partitions										
Throw Away Outdated Newspapers, Magazines, Papers										
Check For Broken Furniture (Report/Schedule Maintenance)										
Light Bulbs Checked And None Functioning Bulbs Replaced										
Check Hardware, Door Stops And Lock Mechanisms										
Fire Exit Lights And Emergency Lights Checked & Functioning										
Test Carbon Monoxide Alarm And Replace Batteries If Required										
Test Smoke Detector Alarm And Replace Batteries If Required										
Paper Dispensers And Paper Towel Rolls Re-Stocked										
Soap Dispensers, Hand Sanitizers And Hand Gels Are Refilled										
Face Masks, Protective Gloves And Face Shields Re-Stocked										

CARE HOME TOILET & RESTROOM CLEANING *Checklist*

Building	Location	Room Number	Area

Start Date & Time	Finnish Date & Time	Name	Signature

	Care Home Cleaning Tasks - Toilet & Restroom	M	T	W	T	F	S	S	Cleaned By	Checked By	Date/Tim
1	Clean And Sanitize All The Counter Tops And Surface Areas										
2	Wipe Down The Walls Wherever There Are Spills And Splashes										
3	Disinfect Touch Points, Light Switches And Other Switches										
4	Clean And Disinfect All Doors, Handles And Doorknobs										
5	Clean And Dust Door Frames, Remember To Dust The Tops										
6	Dust Light Fixtures With A Duster Or A Microfibre Cloth										
7	Wall Mirrors Cleaned With Glass Cleaner										
8	Clean Any Bathroom Glasses And Cups										
9	Clean And Sanitize Any Chairs And Seats										
10	Empty The Waste Basket And Recycling Bin										
11	Clean And Disinfectant The Waste Bin And Recycling Bin										
12	Clean And Wipe Down Windowsills										
13	Spray Air Freshener This Keeps The Room Smelling Fresh										
14	Air/Odour Control Systems Are Filled And Operating Correctly										
15	Clean Skirting Boards/Baseboards And Corners										
16	Vacuum And Hoover Bath Mats, Shower Mats And Rugs										
17	Replace Bath Mats, Shower Mats And Rugs With Clean Ones										
18	Steam Clean Carpets And Rugs										
19	Hand Towels Replaced With Fresh Clean Ones										
20	Bath Towels Replaced With Fresh Clean Ones										
21	Face Towels Replaced With Fresh Clean Ones										
22	Electric Hand Dryers Cleaned, Disinfected & Operating Correctly										
23	Soap Dispensers, Sanitizers And Hand Gels Are Refilled										
24	Clean & Check Contents Of Medicine Trolleys & Cupboards										
25	Clean And Disinfect Any Handrails										
26	Sinks, Taps And Fixtures Cleaned And Disinfected										
27	Clean And Disinfect Cabinets And Units										
28	Feminine Hygiene Dispensers Re-Stocked										
29	Feminine Hygiene Bins/Containers Emptied And Cleared										

Care Home Cleaning Tasks - Toilet & Restroom	M	T	W	T	F	S	S	Cleaned By	Checked By	Date/Time
Clean & Vacuum Central Heating Units (Backs Of Radiators)										
Wash And Clean Ceiling Light Covers										
Toilet Roll Holders And Toilet Rolls Re-Stocked										
Toilet Roll Holders Cleaned And Disinfected										
Clean Inside The Toilets And Urinals With Disinfectant										
Toilet Seats Cleaned And Disinfected										
Clean Top Of Toilets Tanks, The Bases And Behind Toilets										
Urinal Handles Cleaned And Disinfected										
Urinal Screens Cleaned, Disinfected And Blocks Replaced										
Paper Dispensers And Paper Towel Rolls Re-Stocked										
Paper Dispensers And Paper Towel Roll Cleaned & Disinfected										
The Floors Are Swept And Free From Debris And Litter										
Floors Mopped Clean With Cleaning Or Disinfecting Solution										
Put Up Or Place Wet Floor Signs After Mopping Floors										
Showers And Shower Heads, Cleaned And Disinfected										
Soak Shower Heads										
Clean And Disinfect Glass Shower Doors/Outer Doors										
Clean Soap Scum From Shower Walls										
Clean Blinds (Dust The Blinds With A Damp Microfibre Cloth)										
Clean Curtains (Vacuum On A Low Setting Or Wash If Possible)										
Dust And Wash Radiator Covers										
Clean And Disinfect Commodes Between Each Use										
Clean And Disinfect Shower Chairs Between Each Use										
Bath Hoists Cleaned And Disinfected Between Each Use										
Scrub Tub/Bath, Polish Facets And Taps, Clean & Disinfected										
Toothbrush Holders And Soap Holders Cleaned										
Re-Place Shower Curtains With Clean Fresh Ones										
Wash And Clean Air Vents										
Thoroughly Clean Grout And Tiles										
Disinfect And Clean All The Walls From Top To Bottom										
Wash And Clean Windows (Inside And Outside)										
Unclog The Drains (Sink, Bath And Shower)										
Pour Drain Cleaner Down Sink, Shower & Bath Drains										
Floor Drains And Drain Covers Are Open And Free Of Debris										
Hair Dryers Cleaned And Disinfected And Operating Correctly										
Light Bulbs Checked And None Functioning Bulbs Replaced										
Check Hardware, Door Stops And Lock Mechanisms										

CARE HOME BEDROOM CLEANING *Checklist*

Building	Location	Room Number	Area

Start Date & Time	Finnish Date & Time	Name	Signature

	Care Home Cleaning Tasks - Bedrooms	M	T	W	T	F	S	S	Cleaned By	Checked By	Date/Ti
1	Clean And Sanitize All The Desks And Tables										
2	Clean And Sanitize All The Counter Tops And Surface Areas										
3	Wipe Down The Walls Wherever There Are Spills And Splashes										
4	Disinfect Touch Points, Light Switches And Other Switches										
5	Clean And Disinfect All Doors, Handles And Doorknobs										
6	Clean And Dust Door Frames, Remember To Dust The Tops										
7	Dust Light Fixtures With A Duster Or A Microfibre Cloth										
8	Clean & Wipe Mirrors Remove Fingerprints, Smears & Dirt										
9	Clean And Dust Bedside Cabinets										
10	Clean And Sanitize Over Chair Tables										
11	Clean And Sanitize Over Bed Tables										
12	Clean And Check Bed Frames										
13	Mattresses Hoovered And Cleaned With Disinfectant										
14	Clean And Polish Bookshelves, Remember To Dust The Top										
15	Remove, Wash And Clean Any Dirty Cups Or Glasses										
16	Remove, Wash And Clean Any Dirty Plates, Bowels Or Cutlery										
17	Clean And Sanitize Any Chairs And Seats										
18	Water Jug (Washed Thoroughly Each Day & Re-Filled)										
19	Water Any Plants And Flowers										
20	Dust Plant Leafs (A Healthy Plant Needs To Be Clear Of Dust)										
21	Empty The Waste Basket And Recycling Bin										
22	Clean And Disinfectant The Waste Bin And Recycling Bin										
23	Clean And Wipe Down Windowsills										
24	Spray Air Freshener This Keeps The Room Smelling Fresh										
25	Clean And Disinfect Cabinets And Units										
26	Clean And Sanitize Desk Accessories										
27	Replace Dirty Linen And Move To Laundry Room										
28	Polish Any Wooden Furniture And Hardwood Surfaces										
29	Clean Skirting Boards/Baseboards And Corners										

Care Home Cleaning Tasks - Bedrooms Continued	M	T	W	T	F	S	S	Cleaned By	Checked By	Date/Time
Dust Television, Top Sides And Back, TV Unit And TV Stand										
Clean TV Screen With Soft Damp Cloth (Use Water/Cleaner)										
Vacuum/Hoover Between Bedroom Furniture And The Walls										
Clean And Sanitize Resident's Personal Wheelchair										
Check For Broken Wheelchairs, Frames and Wheels										
Vacuum Under Furniture, Beds, Sofas and Dressers										
Vacuum And Hoover The Carpets, Mats And Rugs										
Vacuum Furnishings, Cushions, Chairs, Sofas And Couches										
Steam Clean Carpets And Rugs										
Dust And Clean Any Picture Frames And Photo Frames										
Ledges, Flat Surfaces And The Tops Of Wardrobes Dusted										
Clean & Check Contents Of Medicine Trolleys & Cupboards										
Clean And Sanitize Mobile Phone, Phone Case And Screen										
Clean & Vacuum The Desk Chair, Legs And Chair Wheels										
Wash And Clean Air Vents										
Dust Ceiling Fan Blades With Duster Or A Microfibre Cloth										
Wash And Clean Windows (Inside And Outside)										
Dust And Clean The Walls From Top To Bottom										
Clean Blinds (Dust The Blinds With A Damp Microfibre Cloth)										
Clean Curtains (Vacuum On A Low Setting Or Wash If Possible)										
Dust And Wash Radiator Covers										
Wash And Clean Ceiling Light Covers										
Clean & Vacuum Central Heating Units (Backs Of Radiators)										
Clean And Disinfect Any Handrails										
Hand Towels Replaced With Fresh Clean Ones										
Sink Wall Mirror Cleaned With Glass Cleaner										
Sinks, Taps And Fixtures Cleaned And Disinfected										
Pour Drain Cleaner Down Sink Drains										
Check For Broken Furniture (Report/Schedule Maintenance)										
Light Bulbs Checked And None Functioning Bulbs Replaced										
Check Hardware, Door Stops And Lock Mechanisms										
Fire Exit Lights And Emergency Lights Checked & Functioning										
Test Carbon Monoxide Alarm And Replace Batteries If Required										
Test Smoke Detector Alarm And Replace Batteries If Required										
Paper Dispensers And Paper Towel Rolls Re-Stocked										
Soap Dispensers, Hand Sanitizers And Hand Gels Are Refilled										
Face Masks, Protective Gloves And Face Shields Re-Stocked										

CARE HOME COMMUNAL AREA CLEANING *Checklist*

Building	Location	Room Number	Area

Start Date & Time	Finnish Date & Time	Name	Signature

	Care Home Cleaning Tasks - Communal Area	M	T	W	T	F	S	S	Cleaned By	Checked By	Date/Ti
1	Clean And Sanitize All The Desks And Tables										
2	Clean And Sanitize All The Counter Tops And Surface Areas										
3	Wipe Down The Walls Wherever There Are Spills And Splashes										
4	Disinfect Touch Points, Light Switches And Other Switches										
5	Clean And Disinfect All Doors, Handles And Doorknobs										
6	Clean And Dust Door Frames, Remember To Dust The Tops										
7	Dust Light Fixtures & Shades With A Duster Or A Microfibre Cloth										
8	Clean And Wipe Mirrors Remove Fingerprints, Smears & Dirt										
9	Clean And Sanitize Over Chair Tables										
10	Clean And Polish Bookshelves, Remember To Dust The Top										
11	Remove, Wash And Clean Any Dirty Cups Or Glasses										
12	Remove, Wash And Clean Any Dirty Plates, Bowels Or Cutlery										
13	Clean And Sanitize Any Chairs, Seats And Benches										
14	Water Jugs (Washed Thoroughly Each Day & Re-Filled)										
15	Water Any Plants And Flowers										
16	Dust Plant Leafs (A Healthy Plant Needs To Be Clear Of Dust)										
17	Empty The Waste Baskets And Recycling Bins										
18	Clean And Disinfectant The Waste Bins And Recycling Bins										
19	Clean And Wipe Down Windowsills										
20	Spray Air Freshener This Keeps The Room Smelling Fresh										
21	Clean And Disinfect Cabinets And Units										
22	Clean And Sanitize Desk Accessories										
23	Replace Dirty Table Linen And Move To Laundry Room										
24	Polish Any Wooden Furniture And Hardwood Surfaces										
25	Clean Skirting Boards/Baseboards And Corners										
26	Clean And Polish Fireplace Mantelpiece And Surrounds										
27	Wipe Down Equipment & Sanitize Tea And Coffee Making Facilities										
28	Clean And Sanitize Telephones, Cords/Leads & All Touch Points										
29	Clean And Sanitize Walking Sticks And Any Other Walking Aids										

Care Home Cleaning Tasks - Communal Area	M	T	W	T	F	S	S	Cleaned By	Checked By	Date/Time
Dust Television, Top Sides And Back, TV Unit And TV Stand										
Clean TV Screen With Soft Damp Cloth (Use Water/Cleaner)										
Vacuum/Hoover Between Furniture And The Walls										
Clean And Sanitize All Wheelchairs										
Check For Broken Wheelchairs, Frames and Wheels										
Vacuum Under Furniture, Units, Tables And Cabinets										
Vacuum And Hoover The Carpets, Mats And Rugs										
Vacuum Furnishings, Cushions, Chairs, Sofas And Couches										
Steam Clean Carpets And Rugs										
Dust And Clean Any Picture Frames And Wall Art										
Clean & Check Contents Of Medicine Trolleys & Cupboards										
Clean & Vacuum The Desk Chair, Legs And Chair Wheels										
Wash And Clean Air Vents										
Dust Ceiling Fan Blades With Duster Or A Microfibre Cloth										
Wash And Clean Windows (Inside And Outside)										
Dust And Clean The Walls From Top To Bottom										
Clean Blinds (Dust The Blinds With A Damp Microfibre Cloth)										
Clean Curtains (Vacuum On A Low Setting Or Wash If Possible)										
Dust And Wash Radiator Covers										
Wash And Clean Ceiling Light Covers										
Clean & Vacuum Central Heating Units (Backs Of Radiators)										
Clean And Disinfect Any Handrails										
Clean And Sanitize Computer, Keyboard And Computer Mice										
Clean And Sanitize iPads, Tablets, Laptops & Mobile Phones										
Floors Mopped Clean With Cleaning Or Disinfecting Solution										
The Floors Are Swept And Free From Debris And Litter										
Clean Sliding Doors and Room Partitions										
Throw Away Outdated Newspapers, Magazines, Papers										
Check For Broken Furniture (Report/Schedule Maintenance)										
Light Bulbs Checked And None Functioning Bulbs Replaced										
Check Hardware, Door Stops And Lock Mechanisms										
Fire Exit Lights And Emergency Lights Checked & Functioning										
Test Carbon Monoxide Alarm And Replace Batteries If Required										
Test Smoke Detector Alarm And Replace Batteries If Required										
Paper Dispensers And Paper Towel Rolls Re-Stocked										
Soap Dispensers, Hand Sanitizers And Hand Gels Are Refilled										
Face Masks, Protective Gloves And Face Shields Re-Stocked										

CARE HOME TOILET & RESTROOM CLEANING *Checklist*

Building	Location	Room Number	Area

Start Date & Time	Finnish Date & Time	Name	Signature

	Care Home Cleaning Tasks - Toilet & Restroom	M	T	W	T	F	S	S	Cleaned By	Checked By	Date/Ti
1	Clean And Sanitize All The Counter Tops And Surface Areas										
2	Wipe Down The Walls Wherever There Are Spills And Splashes										
3	Disinfect Touch Points, Light Switches And Other Switches										
4	Clean And Disinfect All Doors, Handles And Doorknobs										
5	Clean And Dust Door Frames, Remember To Dust The Tops										
6	Dust Light Fixtures With A Duster Or A Microfibre Cloth										
7	Wall Mirrors Cleaned With Glass Cleaner										
8	Clean Any Bathroom Glasses And Cups										
9	Clean And Sanitize Any Chairs And Seats										
10	Empty The Waste Basket And Recycling Bin										
11	Clean And Disinfectant The Waste Bin And Recycling Bin										
12	Clean And Wipe Down Windowsills										
13	Spray Air Freshener This Keeps The Room Smelling Fresh										
14	Air/Odour Control Systems Are Filled And Operating Correctly										
15	Clean Skirting Boards/Baseboards And Corners										
16	Vacuum And Hoover Bath Mats, Shower Mats And Rugs										
17	Replace Bath Mats, Shower Mats And Rugs With Clean Ones										
18	Steam Clean Carpets And Rugs										
19	Hand Towels Replaced With Fresh Clean Ones										
20	Bath Towels Replaced With Fresh Clean Ones										
21	Face Towels Replaced With Fresh Clean Ones										
22	Electric Hand Dryers Cleaned, Disinfected & Operating Correctly										
23	Soap Dispensers, Sanitizers And Hand Gels Are Refilled										
24	Clean & Check Contents Of Medicine Trolleys & Cupboards										
25	Clean And Disinfect Any Handrails										
26	Sinks, Taps And Fixtures Cleaned And Disinfected										
27	Clean And Disinfect Cabinets And Units										
28	Feminine Hygiene Dispensers Re-Stocked										
29	Feminine Hygiene Bins/Containers Emptied And Cleared										

Care Home Cleaning Tasks - Toilet & Restroom	M	T	W	T	F	S	S	Cleaned By	Checked By	Date/Time
Clean & Vacuum Central Heating Units (Backs Of Radiators)										
Wash And Clean Ceiling Light Covers										
Toilet Roll Holders And Toilet Rolls Re-Stocked										
Toilet Roll Holders Cleaned And Disinfected										
Clean Inside The Toilets And Urinals With Disinfectant										
Toilet Seats Cleaned And Disinfected										
Clean Top Of Toilets Tanks, The Bases And Behind Toilets										
Urinal Handles Cleaned And Disinfected										
Urinal Screens Cleaned, Disinfected And Blocks Replaced										
Paper Dispensers And Paper Towel Rolls Re-Stocked										
Paper Dispensers And Paper Towel Roll Cleaned & Disinfected										
The Floors Are Swept And Free From Debris And Litter										
Floors Mopped Clean With Cleaning Or Disinfecting Solution										
Put Up Or Place Wet Floor Signs After Mopping Floors										
Showers And Shower Heads, Cleaned And Disinfected										
Soak Shower Heads										
Clean And Disinfect Glass Shower Doors/Outer Doors										
Clean Soap Scum From Shower Walls										
Clean Blinds (Dust The Blinds With A Damp Microfibre Cloth)										
Clean Curtains (Vacuum On A Low Setting Or Wash If Possible)										
Dust And Wash Radiator Covers										
Clean And Disinfect Commodes Between Each Use										
Clean And Disinfect Shower Chairs Between Each Use										
Bath Hoists Cleaned And Disinfected Between Each Use										
Scrub Tub/Bath, Polish Facets And Taps, Clean & Disinfected										
Toothbrush Holders And Soap Holders Cleaned										
Re-Place Shower Curtains With Clean Fresh Ones										
Wash And Clean Air Vents										
Thoroughly Clean Grout And Tiles										
Disinfect And Clean All The Walls From Top To Bottom										
Wash And Clean Windows (Inside And Outside)										
Unclog The Drains (Sink, Bath And Shower)										
Pour Drain Cleaner Down Sink, Shower & Bath Drains										
Floor Drains And Drain Covers Are Open And Free Of Debris										
Hair Dryers Cleaned And Disinfected And Operating Correctly										
Light Bulbs Checked And None Functioning Bulbs Replaced										
Check Hardware, Door Stops And Lock Mechanisms										

CARE HOME BEDROOM CLEANING *Checklist*

Building	Location	Room Number	Area

Start Date & Time	Finnish Date & Time	Name	Signature

	Care Home Cleaning Tasks - Bedrooms	M	T	W	T	F	S	S	Cleaned By	Checked By	Date/Tin
1	Clean And Sanitize All The Desks And Tables										
2	Clean And Sanitize All The Counter Tops And Surface Areas										
3	Wipe Down The Walls Wherever There Are Spills And Splashes										
4	Disinfect Touch Points, Light Switches And Other Switches										
5	Clean And Disinfect All Doors, Handles And Doorknobs										
6	Clean And Dust Door Frames, Remember To Dust The Tops										
7	Dust Light Fixtures With A Duster Or A Microfibre Cloth										
8	Clean & Wipe Mirrors Remove Fingerprints, Smears & Dirt										
9	Clean And Dust Bedside Cabinets										
10	Clean And Sanitize Over Chair Tables										
11	Clean And Sanitize Over Bed Tables										
12	Clean And Check Bed Frames										
13	Mattresses Hoovered And Cleaned With Disinfectant										
14	Clean And Polish Bookshelves, Remember To Dust The Top										
15	Remove, Wash And Clean Any Dirty Cups Or Glasses										
16	Remove, Wash And Clean Any Dirty Plates, Bowels Or Cutlery										
17	Clean And Sanitize Any Chairs And Seats										
18	Water Jug (Washed Thoroughly Each Day & Re-Filled)										
19	Water Any Plants And Flowers										
20	Dust Plant Leafs (A Healthy Plant Needs To Be Clear Of Dust)										
21	Empty The Waste Basket And Recycling Bin										
22	Clean And Disinfectant The Waste Bin And Recycling Bin										
23	Clean And Wipe Down Windowsills										
24	Spray Air Freshener This Keeps The Room Smelling Fresh										
25	Clean And Disinfect Cabinets And Units										
26	Clean And Sanitize Desk Accessories										
27	Replace Dirty Linen And Move To Laundry Room										
28	Polish Any Wooden Furniture And Hardwood Surfaces										
29	Clean Skirting Boards/Baseboards And Corners										

Care Home Cleaning Tasks - Bedrooms Continued	M	T	W	T	F	S	S	Cleaned By	Checked By	Date/Time
Dust Television, Top Sides And Back, TV Unit And TV Stand										
Clean TV Screen With Soft Damp Cloth (Use Water/Cleaner)										
Vacuum/Hoover Between Bedroom Furniture And The Walls										
Clean And Sanitize Resident's Personal Wheelchair										
Check For Broken Wheelchairs, Frames and Wheels										
Vacuum Under Furniture, Beds, Sofas and Dressers										
Vacuum And Hoover The Carpets, Mats And Rugs										
Vacuum Furnishings, Cushions, Chairs, Sofas And Couches										
Steam Clean Carpets And Rugs										
Dust And Clean Any Picture Frames And Photo Frames										
Ledges, Flat Surfaces And The Tops Of Wardrobes Dusted										
Clean & Check Contents Of Medicine Trolleys & Cupboards										
Clean And Sanitize Mobile Phone, Phone Case And Screen										
Clean & Vacuum The Desk Chair, Legs And Chair Wheels										
Wash And Clean Air Vents										
Dust Ceiling Fan Blades With Duster Or A Microfibre Cloth										
Wash And Clean Windows (Inside And Outside)										
Dust And Clean The Walls From Top To Bottom										
Clean Blinds (Dust The Blinds With A Damp Microfibre Cloth)										
Clean Curtains (Vacuum On A Low Setting Or Wash If Possible)										
Dust And Wash Radiator Covers										
Wash And Clean Ceiling Light Covers										
Clean & Vacuum Central Heating Units (Backs Of Radiators)										
Clean And Disinfect Any Handrails										
Hand Towels Replaced With Fresh Clean Ones										
Sink Wall Mirror Cleaned With Glass Cleaner										
Sinks, Taps And Fixtures Cleaned And Disinfected										
Pour Drain Cleaner Down Sink Drains										
Check For Broken Furniture (Report/Schedule Maintenance)										
Light Bulbs Checked And None Functioning Bulbs Replaced										
Check Hardware, Door Stops And Lock Mechanisms										
Fire Exit Lights And Emergency Lights Checked & Functioning										
Test Carbon Monoxide Alarm And Replace Batteries If Required										
Test Smoke Detector Alarm And Replace Batteries If Required										
Paper Dispensers And Paper Towel Rolls Re-Stocked										
Soap Dispensers, Hand Sanitizers And Hand Gels Are Refilled										
Face Masks, Protective Gloves And Face Shields Re-Stocked										

CARE HOME COMMUNAL AREA CLEANING *Checklist*

Building	Location	Room Number	Area

Start Date & Time	Finnish Date & Time	Name	Signature

	Care Home Cleaning Tasks - Communal Area	M	T	W	T	F	S	S	Cleaned By	Checked By	Date/Tin
1	Clean And Sanitize All The Desks And Tables										
2	Clean And Sanitize All The Counter Tops And Surface Areas										
3	Wipe Down The Walls Wherever There Are Spills And Splashes										
4	Disinfect Touch Points, Light Switches And Other Switches										
5	Clean And Disinfect All Doors, Handles And Doorknobs										
6	Clean And Dust Door Frames, Remember To Dust The Tops										
7	Dust Light Fixtures & Shades With A Duster Or A Microfibre Cloth										
8	Clean And Wipe Mirrors Remove Fingerprints, Smears & Dirt										
9	Clean And Sanitize Over Chair Tables										
10	Clean And Polish Bookshelves, Remember To Dust The Top										
11	Remove, Wash And Clean Any Dirty Cups Or Glasses										
12	Remove, Wash And Clean Any Dirty Plates, Bowels Or Cutlery										
13	Clean And Sanitize Any Chairs, Seats And Benches										
14	Water Jugs (Washed Thoroughly Each Day & Re-Filled)										
15	Water Any Plants And Flowers										
16	Dust Plant Leafs (A Healthy Plant Needs To Be Clear Of Dust)										
17	Empty The Waste Baskets And Recycling Bins										
18	Clean And Disinfectant The Waste Bins And Recycling Bins										
19	Clean And Wipe Down Windowsills										
20	Spray Air Freshener This Keeps The Room Smelling Fresh										
21	Clean And Disinfect Cabinets And Units										
22	Clean And Sanitize Desk Accessories										
23	Replace Dirty Table Linen And Move To Laundry Room										
24	Polish Any Wooden Furniture And Hardwood Surfaces										
25	Clean Skirting Boards/Baseboards And Corners										
26	Clean And Polish Fireplace Mantelpiece And Surrounds										
27	Wipe Down Equipment & Sanitize Tea And Coffee Making Facilities										
28	Clean And Sanitize Telephones, Cords/Leads & All Touch Points										
29	Clean And Sanitize Walking Sticks And Any Other Walking Aids										

Care Home Cleaning Tasks - Communal Area	M	T	W	T	F	S	S	Cleaned By	Checked By	Date/Time
Dust Television, Top Sides And Back, TV Unit And TV Stand										
Clean TV Screen With Soft Damp Cloth (Use Water/Cleaner)										
Vacuum/Hoover Between Furniture And The Walls										
Clean And Sanitize All Wheelchairs										
Check For Broken Wheelchairs, Frames and Wheels										
Vacuum Under Furniture, Units, Tables And Cabinets										
Vacuum And Hoover The Carpets, Mats And Rugs										
Vacuum Furnishings, Cushions, Chairs, Sofas And Couches										
Steam Clean Carpets And Rugs										
Dust And Clean Any Picture Frames And Wall Art										
Clean & Check Contents Of Medicine Trolleys & Cupboards										
Clean & Vacuum The Desk Chair, Legs And Chair Wheels										
Wash And Clean Air Vents										
Dust Ceiling Fan Blades With Duster Or A Microfibre Cloth										
Wash And Clean Windows (Inside And Outside)										
Dust And Clean The Walls From Top To Bottom										
Clean Blinds (Dust The Blinds With A Damp Microfibre Cloth)										
Clean Curtains (Vacuum On A Low Setting Or Wash If Possible)										
Dust And Wash Radiator Covers										
Wash And Clean Ceiling Light Covers										
Clean & Vacuum Central Heating Units (Backs Of Radiators)										
Clean And Disinfect Any Handrails										
Clean And Sanitize Computer, Keyboard And Computer Mice										
Clean And Sanitize iPads, Tablets, Laptops & Mobile Phones										
Floors Mopped Clean With Cleaning Or Disinfecting Solution										
The Floors Are Swept And Free From Debris And Litter										
Clean Sliding Doors and Room Partitions										
Throw Away Outdated Newspapers, Magazines, Papers										
Check For Broken Furniture (Report/Schedule Maintenance)										
Light Bulbs Checked And None Functioning Bulbs Replaced										
Check Hardware, Door Stops And Lock Mechanisms										
Fire Exit Lights And Emergency Lights Checked & Functioning										
Test Carbon Monoxide Alarm And Replace Batteries If Required										
Test Smoke Detector Alarm And Replace Batteries If Required										
Paper Dispensers And Paper Towel Rolls Re-Stocked										
Soap Dispensers, Hand Sanitizers And Hand Gels Are Refilled										
Face Masks, Protective Gloves And Face Shields Re-Stocked										

CARE HOME TOILET & RESTROOM CLEANING *Checklist*

Building	Location	Room Number	Area

Start Date & Time	Finnish Date & Time	Name	Signature

	Care Home Cleaning Tasks - Toilet & Restroom	M	T	W	T	F	S	S	Cleaned By	Checked By	Date/Ti
1	Clean And Sanitize All The Counter Tops And Surface Areas										
2	Wipe Down The Walls Wherever There Are Spills And Splashes										
3	Disinfect Touch Points, Light Switches And Other Switches										
4	Clean And Disinfect All Doors, Handles And Doorknobs										
5	Clean And Dust Door Frames, Remember To Dust The Tops										
6	Dust Light Fixtures With A Duster Or A Microfibre Cloth										
7	Wall Mirrors Cleaned With Glass Cleaner										
8	Clean Any Bathroom Glasses And Cups										
9	Clean And Sanitize Any Chairs And Seats										
10	Empty The Waste Basket And Recycling Bin										
11	Clean And Disinfectant The Waste Bin And Recycling Bin										
12	Clean And Wipe Down Windowsills										
13	Spray Air Freshener This Keeps The Room Smelling Fresh										
14	Air/Odour Control Systems Are Filled And Operating Correctly										
15	Clean Skirting Boards/Baseboards And Corners										
16	Vacuum And Hoover Bath Mats, Shower Mats And Rugs										
17	Replace Bath Mats, Shower Mats And Rugs With Clean Ones										
18	Steam Clean Carpets And Rugs										
19	Hand Towels Replaced With Fresh Clean Ones										
20	Bath Towels Replaced With Fresh Clean Ones										
21	Face Towels Replaced With Fresh Clean Ones										
22	Electric Hand Dryers Cleaned, Disinfected & Operating Correctly										
23	Soap Dispensers, Sanitizers And Hand Gels Are Refilled										
24	Clean & Check Contents Of Medicine Trolleys & Cupboards										
25	Clean And Disinfect Any Handrails										
26	Sinks, Taps And Fixtures Cleaned And Disinfected										
27	Clean And Disinfect Cabinets And Units										
28	Feminine Hygiene Dispensers Re-Stocked										
29	Feminine Hygiene Bins/Containers Emptied And Cleared										

Care Home Cleaning Tasks - Toilet & Restroom	M	T	W	T	F	S	S	Cleaned By	Checked By	Date/Time
Clean & Vacuum Central Heating Units (Backs Of Radiators)										
Wash And Clean Ceiling Light Covers										
Toilet Roll Holders And Toilet Rolls Re-Stocked										
Toilet Roll Holders Cleaned And Disinfected										
Clean Inside The Toilets And Urinals With Disinfectant										
Toilet Seats Cleaned And Disinfected										
Clean Top Of Toilets Tanks, The Bases And Behind Toilets										
Urinal Handles Cleaned And Disinfected										
Urinal Screens Cleaned, Disinfected And Blocks Replaced										
Paper Dispensers And Paper Towel Rolls Re-Stocked										
Paper Dispensers And Paper Towel Roll Cleaned & Disinfected										
The Floors Are Swept And Free From Debris And Litter										
Floors Mopped Clean With Cleaning Or Disinfecting Solution										
Put Up Or Place Wet Floor Signs After Mopping Floors										
Showers And Shower Heads, Cleaned And Disinfected										
Soak Shower Heads										
Clean And Disinfect Glass Shower Doors/Outer Doors										
Clean Soap Scum From Shower Walls										
Clean Blinds (Dust The Blinds With A Damp Microfibre Cloth)										
Clean Curtains (Vacuum On A Low Setting Or Wash If Possible)										
Dust And Wash Radiator Covers										
Clean And Disinfect Commodes Between Each Use										
Clean And Disinfect Shower Chairs Between Each Use										
Bath Hoists Cleaned And Disinfected Between Each Use										
Scrub Tub/Bath, Polish Facets And Taps, Clean & Disinfected										
Toothbrush Holders And Soap Holders Cleaned										
Re-Place Shower Curtains With Clean Fresh Ones										
Wash And Clean Air Vents										
Thoroughly Clean Grout And Tiles										
Disinfect And Clean All The Walls From Top To Bottom										
Wash And Clean Windows (Inside And Outside)										
Unclog The Drains (Sink, Bath And Shower)										
Pour Drain Cleaner Down Sink, Shower & Bath Drains										
Floor Drains And Drain Covers Are Open And Free Of Debris										
Hair Dryers Cleaned And Disinfected And Operating Correctly										
Light Bulbs Checked And None Functioning Bulbs Replaced										
Check Hardware, Door Stops And Lock Mechanisms										

CARE HOME BEDROOM CLEANING *Checklist*

Building	Location	Room Number	Area

Start Date & Time	Finnish Date & Time	Name	Signature

	Care Home Cleaning Tasks - Bedrooms	M	T	W	T	F	S	S	Cleaned By	Checked By	Date/Ti
1	Clean And Sanitize All The Desks And Tables										
2	Clean And Sanitize All The Counter Tops And Surface Areas										
3	Wipe Down The Walls Wherever There Are Spills And Splashes										
4	Disinfect Touch Points, Light Switches And Other Switches										
5	Clean And Disinfect All Doors, Handles And Doorknobs										
6	Clean And Dust Door Frames, Remember To Dust The Tops										
7	Dust Light Fixtures With A Duster Or A Microfibre Cloth										
8	Clean & Wipe Mirrors Remove Fingerprints, Smears & Dirt										
9	Clean And Dust Bedside Cabinets										
10	Clean And Sanitize Over Chair Tables										
11	Clean And Sanitize Over Bed Tables										
12	Clean And Check Bed Frames										
13	Mattresses Hoovered And Cleaned With Disinfectant										
14	Clean And Polish Bookshelves, Remember To Dust The Top										
15	Remove, Wash And Clean Any Dirty Cups Or Glasses										
16	Remove, Wash And Clean Any Dirty Plates, Bowels Or Cutlery										
17	Clean And Sanitize Any Chairs And Seats										
18	Water Jug (Washed Thoroughly Each Day & Re-Filled)										
19	Water Any Plants And Flowers										
20	Dust Plant Leafs (A Healthy Plant Needs To Be Clear Of Dust)										
21	Empty The Waste Basket And Recycling Bin										
22	Clean And Disinfectant The Waste Bin And Recycling Bin										
23	Clean And Wipe Down Windowsills										
24	Spray Air Freshener This Keeps The Room Smelling Fresh										
25	Clean And Disinfect Cabinets And Units										
26	Clean And Sanitize Desk Accessories										
27	Replace Dirty Linen And Move To Laundry Room										
28	Polish Any Wooden Furniture And Hardwood Surfaces										
29	Clean Skirting Boards/Baseboards And Corners										

Care Home Cleaning Tasks - Bedrooms Continued	M	T	W	T	F	S	S	Cleaned By	Checked By	Date/Time
Dust Television, Top Sides And Back, TV Unit And TV Stand										
Clean TV Screen With Soft Damp Cloth (Use Water/Cleaner)										
Vacuum/Hoover Between Bedroom Furniture And The Walls										
Clean And Sanitize Resident's Personal Wheelchair										
Check For Broken Wheelchairs, Frames and Wheels										
Vacuum Under Furniture, Beds, Sofas and Dressers										
Vacuum And Hoover The Carpets, Mats And Rugs										
Vacuum Furnishings, Cushions, Chairs, Sofas And Couches										
Steam Clean Carpets And Rugs										
Dust And Clean Any Picture Frames And Photo Frames										
Ledges, Flat Surfaces And The Tops Of Wardrobes Dusted										
Clean & Check Contents Of Medicine Trolleys & Cupboards										
Clean And Sanitize Mobile Phone, Phone Case And Screen										
Clean & Vacuum The Desk Chair, Legs And Chair Wheels										
Wash And Clean Air Vents										
Dust Ceiling Fan Blades With Duster Or A Microfibre Cloth										
Wash And Clean Windows (Inside And Outside)										
Dust And Clean The Walls From Top To Bottom										
Clean Blinds (Dust The Blinds With A Damp Microfibre Cloth)										
Clean Curtains (Vacuum On A Low Setting Or Wash If Possible)										
Dust And Wash Radiator Covers										
Wash And Clean Ceiling Light Covers										
Clean & Vacuum Central Heating Units (Backs Of Radiators)										
Clean And Disinfect Any Handrails										
Hand Towels Replaced With Fresh Clean Ones										
Sink Wall Mirror Cleaned With Glass Cleaner										
Sinks, Taps And Fixtures Cleaned And Disinfected										
Pour Drain Cleaner Down Sink Drains										
Check For Broken Furniture (Report/Schedule Maintenance)										
Light Bulbs Checked And None Functioning Bulbs Replaced										
Check Hardware, Door Stops And Lock Mechanisms										
Fire Exit Lights And Emergency Lights Checked & Functioning										
Test Carbon Monoxide Alarm And Replace Batteries If Required										
Test Smoke Detector Alarm And Replace Batteries If Required										
Paper Dispensers And Paper Towel Rolls Re-Stocked										
Soap Dispensers, Hand Sanitizers And Hand Gels Are Refilled										
Face Masks, Protective Gloves And Face Shields Re-Stocked										

CARE HOME COMMUNAL AREA CLEANING *Checklist*

Building	Location	Room Number	Area

Start Date & Time	Finnish Date & Time	Name	Signature

	Care Home Cleaning Tasks - Communal Area	M	T	W	T	F	S	S	Cleaned By	Checked By	Date/Tim
1	Clean And Sanitize All The Desks And Tables										
2	Clean And Sanitize All The Counter Tops And Surface Areas										
3	Wipe Down The Walls Wherever There Are Spills And Splashes										
4	Disinfect Touch Points, Light Switches And Other Switches										
5	Clean And Disinfect All Doors, Handles And Doorknobs										
6	Clean And Dust Door Frames, Remember To Dust The Tops										
7	Dust Light Fixtures & Shades With A Duster Or A Microfibre Cloth										
8	Clean And Wipe Mirrors Remove Fingerprints, Smears & Dirt										
9	Clean And Sanitize Over Chair Tables										
10	Clean And Polish Bookshelves, Remember To Dust The Top										
11	Remove, Wash And Clean Any Dirty Cups Or Glasses										
12	Remove, Wash And Clean Any Dirty Plates, Bowels Or Cutlery										
13	Clean And Sanitize Any Chairs, Seats And Benches										
14	Water Jugs (Washed Thoroughly Each Day & Re-Filled)										
15	Water Any Plants And Flowers										
16	Dust Plant Leafs (A Healthy Plant Needs To Be Clear Of Dust)										
17	Empty The Waste Baskets And Recycling Bins										
18	Clean And Disinfectant The Waste Bins And Recycling Bins										
19	Clean And Wipe Down Windowsills										
20	Spray Air Freshener This Keeps The Room Smelling Fresh										
21	Clean And Disinfect Cabinets And Units										
22	Clean And Sanitize Desk Accessories										
23	Replace Dirty Table Linen And Move To Laundry Room										
24	Polish Any Wooden Furniture And Hardwood Surfaces										
25	Clean Skirting Boards/Baseboards And Corners										
26	Clean And Polish Fireplace Mantelpiece And Surrounds										
27	Wipe Down Equipment & Sanitize Tea And Coffee Making Facilities										
28	Clean And Sanitize Telephones, Cords/Leads & All Touch Points										
29	Clean And Sanitize Walking Sticks And Any Other Walking Aids										

Care Home Cleaning Tasks - Communal Area	M	T	W	T	F	S	S	Cleaned By	Checked By	Date/Time
Dust Television, Top Sides And Back, TV Unit And TV Stand										
Clean TV Screen With Soft Damp Cloth (Use Water/Cleaner)										
Vacuum/Hoover Between Furniture And The Walls										
Clean And Sanitize All Wheelchairs										
Check For Broken Wheelchairs, Frames and Wheels										
Vacuum Under Furniture, Units, Tables And Cabinets										
Vacuum And Hoover The Carpets, Mats And Rugs										
Vacuum Furnishings, Cushions, Chairs, Sofas And Couches										
Steam Clean Carpets And Rugs										
Dust And Clean Any Picture Frames And Wall Art										
Clean & Check Contents Of Medicine Trolleys & Cupboards										
Clean & Vacuum The Desk Chair, Legs And Chair Wheels										
Wash And Clean Air Vents										
Dust Ceiling Fan Blades With Duster Or A Microfibre Cloth										
Wash And Clean Windows (Inside And Outside)										
Dust And Clean The Walls From Top To Bottom										
Clean Blinds (Dust The Blinds With A Damp Microfibre Cloth)										
Clean Curtains (Vacuum On A Low Setting Or Wash If Possible)										
Dust And Wash Radiator Covers										
Wash And Clean Ceiling Light Covers										
Clean & Vacuum Central Heating Units (Backs Of Radiators)										
Clean And Disinfect Any Handrails										
Clean And Sanitize Computer, Keyboard And Computer Mice										
Clean And Sanitize iPads, Tablets, Laptops & Mobile Phones										
Floors Mopped Clean With Cleaning Or Disinfecting Solution										
The Floors Are Swept And Free From Debris And Litter										
Clean Sliding Doors and Room Partitions										
Throw Away Outdated Newspapers, Magazines, Papers										
Check For Broken Furniture (Report/Schedule Maintenance)										
Light Bulbs Checked And None Functioning Bulbs Replaced										
Check Hardware, Door Stops And Lock Mechanisms										
Fire Exit Lights And Emergency Lights Checked & Functioning										
Test Carbon Monoxide Alarm And Replace Batteries If Required										
Test Smoke Detector Alarm And Replace Batteries If Required										
Paper Dispensers And Paper Towel Rolls Re-Stocked										
Soap Dispensers, Hand Sanitizers And Hand Gels Are Refilled										
Face Masks, Protective Gloves And Face Shields Re-Stocked										

CARE HOME TOILET & RESTROOM CLEANING *Checklist*

Building	Location	Room Number	Area

Start Date & Time	Finnish Date & Time	Name	Signature

	Care Home Cleaning Tasks - Toilet & Restroom	M	T	W	T	F	S	S	Cleaned By	Checked By	Date/Ti
1	Clean And Sanitize All The Counter Tops And Surface Areas										
2	Wipe Down The Walls Wherever There Are Spills And Splashes										
3	Disinfect Touch Points, Light Switches And Other Switches										
4	Clean And Disinfect All Doors, Handles And Doorknobs										
5	Clean And Dust Door Frames, Remember To Dust The Tops										
6	Dust Light Fixtures With A Duster Or A Microfibre Cloth										
7	Wall Mirrors Cleaned With Glass Cleaner										
8	Clean Any Bathroom Glasses And Cups										
9	Clean And Sanitize Any Chairs And Seats										
10	Empty The Waste Basket And Recycling Bin										
11	Clean And Disinfectant The Waste Bin And Recycling Bin										
12	Clean And Wipe Down Windowsills										
13	Spray Air Freshener This Keeps The Room Smelling Fresh										
14	Air/Odour Control Systems Are Filled And Operating Correctly										
15	Clean Skirting Boards/Baseboards And Corners										
16	Vacuum And Hoover Bath Mats, Shower Mats And Rugs										
17	Replace Bath Mats, Shower Mats And Rugs With Clean Ones										
18	Steam Clean Carpets And Rugs										
19	Hand Towels Replaced With Fresh Clean Ones										
20	Bath Towels Replaced With Fresh Clean Ones										
21	Face Towels Replaced With Fresh Clean Ones										
22	Electric Hand Dryers Cleaned, Disinfected & Operating Correctly										
23	Soap Dispensers, Sanitizers And Hand Gels Are Refilled										
24	Clean & Check Contents Of Medicine Trolleys & Cupboards										
25	Clean And Disinfect Any Handrails										
26	Sinks, Taps And Fixtures Cleaned And Disinfected										
27	Clean And Disinfect Cabinets And Units										
28	Feminine Hygiene Dispensers Re-Stocked										
29	Feminine Hygiene Bins/Containers Emptied And Cleared										

Care Home Cleaning Tasks - Toilet & Restroom	M	T	W	T	F	S	S	Cleaned By	Checked By	Date/Time
Clean & Vacuum Central Heating Units (Backs Of Radiators)										
Wash And Clean Ceiling Light Covers										
Toilet Roll Holders And Toilet Rolls Re-Stocked										
Toilet Roll Holders Cleaned And Disinfected										
Clean Inside The Toilets And Urinals With Disinfectant										
Toilet Seats Cleaned And Disinfected										
Clean Top Of Toilets Tanks, The Bases And Behind Toilets										
Urinal Handles Cleaned And Disinfected										
Urinal Screens Cleaned, Disinfected And Blocks Replaced										
Paper Dispensers And Paper Towel Rolls Re-Stocked										
Paper Dispensers And Paper Towel Roll Cleaned & Disinfected										
The Floors Are Swept And Free From Debris And Litter										
Floors Mopped Clean With Cleaning Or Disinfecting Solution										
Put Up Or Place Wet Floor Signs After Mopping Floors										
Showers And Shower Heads, Cleaned And Disinfected										
Soak Shower Heads										
Clean And Disinfect Glass Shower Doors/Outer Doors										
Clean Soap Scum From Shower Walls										
Clean Blinds (Dust The Blinds With A Damp Microfibre Cloth)										
Clean Curtains (Vacuum On A Low Setting Or Wash If Possible)										
Dust And Wash Radiator Covers										
Clean And Disinfect Commodes Between Each Use										
Clean And Disinfect Shower Chairs Between Each Use										
Bath Hoists Cleaned And Disinfected Between Each Use										
Scrub Tub/Bath, Polish Facets And Taps, Clean & Disinfected										
Toothbrush Holders And Soap Holders Cleaned										
Re-Place Shower Curtains With Clean Fresh Ones										
Wash And Clean Air Vents										
Thoroughly Clean Grout And Tiles										
Disinfect And Clean All The Walls From Top To Bottom										
Wash And Clean Windows (Inside And Outside)										
Unclog The Drains (Sink, Bath And Shower)										
Pour Drain Cleaner Down Sink, Shower & Bath Drains										
Floor Drains And Drain Covers Are Open And Free Of Debris										
Hair Dryers Cleaned And Disinfected And Operating Correctly										
Light Bulbs Checked And None Functioning Bulbs Replaced										
Check Hardware, Door Stops And Lock Mechanisms										

CARE HOME BEDROOM CLEANING *Checklist*

Building	Location	Room Number	Area

Start Date & Time	Finnish Date & Time	Name	Signature

	Care Home Cleaning Tasks - Bedrooms	M	T	W	T	F	S	S	Cleaned By	Checked By	Date/Ti
1	Clean And Sanitize All The Desks And Tables										
2	Clean And Sanitize All The Counter Tops And Surface Areas										
3	Wipe Down The Walls Wherever There Are Spills And Splashes										
4	Disinfect Touch Points, Light Switches And Other Switches										
5	Clean And Disinfect All Doors, Handles And Doorknobs										
6	Clean And Dust Door Frames, Remember To Dust The Tops										
7	Dust Light Fixtures With A Duster Or A Microfibre Cloth										
8	Clean & Wipe Mirrors Remove Fingerprints, Smears & Dirt										
9	Clean And Dust Bedside Cabinets										
10	Clean And Sanitize Over Chair Tables										
11	Clean And Sanitize Over Bed Tables										
12	Clean And Check Bed Frames										
13	Mattresses Hoovered And Cleaned With Disinfectant										
14	Clean And Polish Bookshelves, Remember To Dust The Top										
15	Remove, Wash And Clean Any Dirty Cups Or Glasses										
16	Remove, Wash And Clean Any Dirty Plates, Bowels Or Cutlery										
17	Clean And Sanitize Any Chairs And Seats										
18	Water Jug (Washed Thoroughly Each Day & Re-Filled)										
19	Water Any Plants And Flowers										
20	Dust Plant Leafs (A Healthy Plant Needs To Be Clear Of Dust)										
21	Empty The Waste Basket And Recycling Bin										
22	Clean And Disinfectant The Waste Bin And Recycling Bin										
23	Clean And Wipe Down Windowsills										
24	Spray Air Freshener This Keeps The Room Smelling Fresh										
25	Clean And Disinfect Cabinets And Units										
26	Clean And Sanitize Desk Accessories										
27	Replace Dirty Linen And Move To Laundry Room										
28	Polish Any Wooden Furniture And Hardwood Surfaces										
29	Clean Skirting Boards/Baseboards And Corners										

Care Home Cleaning Tasks - Bedrooms Continued	M	T	W	T	F	S	S	Cleaned By	Checked By	Date/Time
Dust Television, Top Sides And Back, TV Unit And TV Stand										
Clean TV Screen With Soft Damp Cloth (Use Water/Cleaner)										
Vacuum/Hoover Between Bedroom Furniture And The Walls										
Clean And Sanitize Resident's Personal Wheelchair										
Check For Broken Wheelchairs, Frames and Wheels										
Vacuum Under Furniture, Beds, Sofas and Dressers										
Vacuum And Hoover The Carpets, Mats And Rugs										
Vacuum Furnishings, Cushions, Chairs, Sofas And Couches										
Steam Clean Carpets And Rugs										
Dust And Clean Any Picture Frames And Photo Frames										
Ledges, Flat Surfaces And The Tops Of Wardrobes Dusted										
Clean & Check Contents Of Medicine Trolleys & Cupboards										
Clean And Sanitize Mobile Phone, Phone Case And Screen										
Clean & Vacuum The Desk Chair, Legs And Chair Wheels										
Wash And Clean Air Vents										
Dust Ceiling Fan Blades With Duster Or A Microfibre Cloth										
Wash And Clean Windows (Inside And Outside)										
Dust And Clean The Walls From Top To Bottom										
Clean Blinds (Dust The Blinds With A Damp Microfibre Cloth)										
Clean Curtains (Vacuum On A Low Setting Or Wash If Possible)										
Dust And Wash Radiator Covers										
Wash And Clean Ceiling Light Covers										
Clean & Vacuum Central Heating Units (Backs Of Radiators)										
Clean And Disinfect Any Handrails										
Hand Towels Replaced With Fresh Clean Ones										
Sink Wall Mirror Cleaned With Glass Cleaner										
Sinks, Taps And Fixtures Cleaned And Disinfected										
Pour Drain Cleaner Down Sink Drains										
Check For Broken Furniture (Report/Schedule Maintenance)										
Light Bulbs Checked And None Functioning Bulbs Replaced										
Check Hardware, Door Stops And Lock Mechanisms										
Fire Exit Lights And Emergency Lights Checked & Functioning										
Test Carbon Monoxide Alarm And Replace Batteries If Required										
Test Smoke Detector Alarm And Replace Batteries If Required										
Paper Dispensers And Paper Towel Rolls Re-Stocked										
Soap Dispensers, Hand Sanitizers And Hand Gels Are Refilled										
Face Masks, Protective Gloves And Face Shields Re-Stocked										

CARE HOME COMMUNAL AREA CLEANING *Checklist*

Building	Location	Room Number	Area

Start Date & Time	Finnish Date & Time	Name	Signature

	Care Home Cleaning Tasks - Communal Area	M	T	W	T	F	S	S	Cleaned By	Checked By	Date/Tim
1	Clean And Sanitize All The Desks And Tables										
2	Clean And Sanitize All The Counter Tops And Surface Areas										
3	Wipe Down The Walls Wherever There Are Spills And Splashes										
4	Disinfect Touch Points, Light Switches And Other Switches										
5	Clean And Disinfect All Doors, Handles And Doorknobs										
6	Clean And Dust Door Frames, Remember To Dust The Tops										
7	Dust Light Fixtures & Shades With A Duster Or A Microfibre Cloth										
8	Clean And Wipe Mirrors Remove Fingerprints, Smears & Dirt										
9	Clean And Sanitize Over Chair Tables										
10	Clean And Polish Bookshelves, Remember To Dust The Top										
11	Remove, Wash And Clean Any Dirty Cups Or Glasses										
12	Remove, Wash And Clean Any Dirty Plates, Bowels Or Cutlery										
13	Clean And Sanitize Any Chairs, Seats And Benches										
14	Water Jugs (Washed Thoroughly Each Day & Re-Filled)										
15	Water Any Plants And Flowers										
16	Dust Plant Leafs (A Healthy Plant Needs To Be Clear Of Dust)										
17	Empty The Waste Baskets And Recycling Bins										
18	Clean And Disinfectant The Waste Bins And Recycling Bins										
19	Clean And Wipe Down Windowsills										
20	Spray Air Freshener This Keeps The Room Smelling Fresh										
21	Clean And Disinfect Cabinets And Units										
22	Clean And Sanitize Desk Accessories										
23	Replace Dirty Table Linen And Move To Laundry Room										
24	Polish Any Wooden Furniture And Hardwood Surfaces										
25	Clean Skirting Boards/Baseboards And Corners										
26	Clean And Polish Fireplace Mantelpiece And Surrounds										
27	Wipe Down Equipment & Sanitize Tea And Coffee Making Facilities										
28	Clean And Sanitize Telephones, Cords/Leads & All Touch Points										
29	Clean And Sanitize Walking Sticks And Any Other Walking Aids										

Care Home Cleaning Tasks - Communal Area	M	T	W	T	F	S	S	Cleaned By	Checked By	Date/Time
Dust Television, Top Sides And Back, TV Unit And TV Stand										
Clean TV Screen With Soft Damp Cloth (Use Water/Cleaner)										
Vacuum/Hoover Between Furniture And The Walls										
Clean And Sanitize All Wheelchairs										
Check For Broken Wheelchairs, Frames and Wheels										
Vacuum Under Furniture, Units, Tables And Cabinets										
Vacuum And Hoover The Carpets, Mats And Rugs										
Vacuum Furnishings, Cushions, Chairs, Sofas And Couches										
Steam Clean Carpets And Rugs										
Dust And Clean Any Picture Frames And Wall Art										
Clean & Check Contents Of Medicine Trolleys & Cupboards										
Clean & Vacuum The Desk Chair, Legs And Chair Wheels										
Wash And Clean Air Vents										
Dust Ceiling Fan Blades With Duster Or A Microfibre Cloth										
Wash And Clean Windows (Inside And Outside)										
Dust And Clean The Walls From Top To Bottom										
Clean Blinds (Dust The Blinds With A Damp Microfibre Cloth)										
Clean Curtains (Vacuum On A Low Setting Or Wash If Possible)										
Dust And Wash Radiator Covers										
Wash And Clean Ceiling Light Covers										
Clean & Vacuum Central Heating Units (Backs Of Radiators)										
Clean And Disinfect Any Handrails										
Clean And Sanitize Computer, Keyboard And Computer Mice										
Clean And Sanitize iPads, Tablets, Laptops & Mobile Phones										
Floors Mopped Clean With Cleaning Or Disinfecting Solution										
The Floors Are Swept And Free From Debris And Litter										
Clean Sliding Doors and Room Partitions										
Throw Away Outdated Newspapers, Magazines, Papers										
Check For Broken Furniture (Report/Schedule Maintenance)										
Light Bulbs Checked And None Functioning Bulbs Replaced										
Check Hardware, Door Stops And Lock Mechanisms										
Fire Exit Lights And Emergency Lights Checked & Functioning										
Test Carbon Monoxide Alarm And Replace Batteries If Required										
Test Smoke Detector Alarm And Replace Batteries If Required										
Paper Dispensers And Paper Towel Rolls Re-Stocked										
Soap Dispensers, Hand Sanitizers And Hand Gels Are Refilled										
Face Masks, Protective Gloves And Face Shields Re-Stocked										

CARE HOME TOILET & RESTROOM CLEANING *Checklist*

Building	Location	Room Number	Area

Start Date & Time	Finnish Date & Time	Name	Signature

	Care Home Cleaning Tasks - Toilet & Restroom	M	T	W	T	F	S	S	Cleaned By	Checked By	Date/Tim
1	Clean And Sanitize All The Counter Tops And Surface Areas										
2	Wipe Down The Walls Wherever There Are Spills And Splashes										
3	Disinfect Touch Points, Light Switches And Other Switches										
4	Clean And Disinfect All Doors, Handles And Doorknobs										
5	Clean And Dust Door Frames, Remember To Dust The Tops										
6	Dust Light Fixtures With A Duster Or A Microfibre Cloth										
7	Wall Mirrors Cleaned With Glass Cleaner										
8	Clean Any Bathroom Glasses And Cups										
9	Clean And Sanitize Any Chairs And Seats										
10	Empty The Waste Basket And Recycling Bin										
11	Clean And Disinfectant The Waste Bin And Recycling Bin										
12	Clean And Wipe Down Windowsills										
13	Spray Air Freshener This Keeps The Room Smelling Fresh										
14	Air/Odour Control Systems Are Filled And Operating Correctly										
15	Clean Skirting Boards/Baseboards And Corners										
16	Vacuum And Hoover Bath Mats, Shower Mats And Rugs										
17	Replace Bath Mats, Shower Mats And Rugs With Clean Ones										
18	Steam Clean Carpets And Rugs										
19	Hand Towels Replaced With Fresh Clean Ones										
20	Bath Towels Replaced With Fresh Clean Ones										
21	Face Towels Replaced With Fresh Clean Ones										
22	Electric Hand Dryers Cleaned, Disinfected & Operating Correctly										
23	Soap Dispensers, Sanitizers And Hand Gels Are Refilled										
24	Clean & Check Contents Of Medicine Trolleys & Cupboards										
25	Clean And Disinfect Any Handrails										
26	Sinks, Taps And Fixtures Cleaned And Disinfected										
27	Clean And Disinfect Cabinets And Units										
28	Feminine Hygiene Dispensers Re-Stocked										
29	Feminine Hygiene Bins/Containers Emptied And Cleared										

Care Home Cleaning Tasks - Toilet & Restroom	M	T	W	T	F	S	S	Cleaned By	Checked By	Date/Time
Clean & Vacuum Central Heating Units (Backs Of Radiators)										
Wash And Clean Ceiling Light Covers										
Toilet Roll Holders And Toilet Rolls Re-Stocked										
Toilet Roll Holders Cleaned And Disinfected										
Clean Inside The Toilets And Urinals With Disinfectant										
Toilet Seats Cleaned And Disinfected										
Clean Top Of Toilets Tanks, The Bases And Behind Toilets										
Urinal Handles Cleaned And Disinfected										
Urinal Screens Cleaned, Disinfected And Blocks Replaced										
Paper Dispensers And Paper Towel Rolls Re-Stocked										
Paper Dispensers And Paper Towel Roll Cleaned & Disinfected										
The Floors Are Swept And Free From Debris And Litter										
Floors Mopped Clean With Cleaning Or Disinfecting Solution										
Put Up Or Place Wet Floor Signs After Mopping Floors										
Showers And Shower Heads, Cleaned And Disinfected										
Soak Shower Heads										
Clean And Disinfect Glass Shower Doors/Outer Doors										
Clean Soap Scum From Shower Walls										
Clean Blinds (Dust The Blinds With A Damp Microfibre Cloth)										
Clean Curtains (Vacuum On A Low Setting Or Wash If Possible)										
Dust And Wash Radiator Covers										
Clean And Disinfect Commodes Between Each Use										
Clean And Disinfect Shower Chairs Between Each Use										
Bath Hoists Cleaned And Disinfected Between Each Use										
Scrub Tub/Bath, Polish Facets And Taps, Clean & Disinfected										
Toothbrush Holders And Soap Holders Cleaned										
Re-Place Shower Curtains With Clean Fresh Ones										
Wash And Clean Air Vents										
Thoroughly Clean Grout And Tiles										
Disinfect And Clean All The Walls From Top To Bottom										
Wash And Clean Windows (Inside And Outside)										
Unclog The Drains (Sink, Bath And Shower)										
Pour Drain Cleaner Down Sink, Shower & Bath Drains										
Floor Drains And Drain Covers Are Open And Free Of Debris										
Hair Dryers Cleaned And Disinfected And Operating Correctly										
Light Bulbs Checked And None Functioning Bulbs Replaced										
Check Hardware, Door Stops And Lock Mechanisms										

CARE HOME BEDROOM CLEANING *Checklist*

Building	Location	Room Number	Area

Start Date & Time	Finnish Date & Time	Name	Signature

	Care Home Cleaning Tasks - Bedrooms	M	T	W	T	F	S	S	Cleaned By	Checked By	Date/Ti
1	Clean And Sanitize All The Desks And Tables										
2	Clean And Sanitize All The Counter Tops And Surface Areas										
3	Wipe Down The Walls Wherever There Are Spills And Splashes										
4	Disinfect Touch Points, Light Switches And Other Switches										
5	Clean And Disinfect All Doors, Handles And Doorknobs										
6	Clean And Dust Door Frames, Remember To Dust The Tops										
7	Dust Light Fixtures With A Duster Or A Microfibre Cloth										
8	Clean & Wipe Mirrors Remove Fingerprints, Smears & Dirt										
9	Clean And Dust Bedside Cabinets										
10	Clean And Sanitize Over Chair Tables										
11	Clean And Sanitize Over Bed Tables										
12	Clean And Check Bed Frames										
13	Mattresses Hoovered And Cleaned With Disinfectant										
14	Clean And Polish Bookshelves, Remember To Dust The Top										
15	Remove, Wash And Clean Any Dirty Cups Or Glasses										
16	Remove, Wash And Clean Any Dirty Plates, Bowels Or Cutlery										
17	Clean And Sanitize Any Chairs And Seats										
18	Water Jug (Washed Thoroughly Each Day & Re-Filled)										
19	Water Any Plants And Flowers										
20	Dust Plant Leafs (A Healthy Plant Needs To Be Clear Of Dust)										
21	Empty The Waste Basket And Recycling Bin										
22	Clean And Disinfectant The Waste Bin And Recycling Bin										
23	Clean And Wipe Down Windowsills										
24	Spray Air Freshener This Keeps The Room Smelling Fresh										
25	Clean And Disinfect Cabinets And Units										
26	Clean And Sanitize Desk Accessories										
27	Replace Dirty Linen And Move To Laundry Room										
28	Polish Any Wooden Furniture And Hardwood Surfaces										
29	Clean Skirting Boards/Baseboards And Corners										

Care Home Cleaning Tasks - Bedrooms Continued	M	T	W	T	F	S	S	Cleaned By	Checked By	Date/Time
Dust Television, Top Sides And Back, TV Unit And TV Stand										
Clean TV Screen With Soft Damp Cloth (Use Water/Cleaner)										
Vacuum/Hoover Between Bedroom Furniture And The Walls										
Clean And Sanitize Resident's Personal Wheelchair										
Check For Broken Wheelchairs, Frames and Wheels										
Vacuum Under Furniture, Beds, Sofas and Dressers										
Vacuum And Hoover The Carpets, Mats And Rugs										
Vacuum Furnishings, Cushions, Chairs, Sofas And Couches										
Steam Clean Carpets And Rugs										
Dust And Clean Any Picture Frames And Photo Frames										
Ledges, Flat Surfaces And The Tops Of Wardrobes Dusted										
Clean & Check Contents Of Medicine Trolleys & Cupboards										
Clean And Sanitize Mobile Phone, Phone Case And Screen										
Clean & Vacuum The Desk Chair, Legs And Chair Wheels										
Wash And Clean Air Vents										
Dust Ceiling Fan Blades With Duster Or A Microfibre Cloth										
Wash And Clean Windows (Inside And Outside)										
Dust And Clean The Walls From Top To Bottom										
Clean Blinds (Dust The Blinds With A Damp Microfibre Cloth)										
Clean Curtains (Vacuum On A Low Setting Or Wash If Possible)										
Dust And Wash Radiator Covers										
Wash And Clean Ceiling Light Covers										
Clean & Vacuum Central Heating Units (Backs Of Radiators)										
Clean And Disinfect Any Handrails										
Hand Towels Replaced With Fresh Clean Ones										
Sink Wall Mirror Cleaned With Glass Cleaner										
Sinks, Taps And Fixtures Cleaned And Disinfected										
Pour Drain Cleaner Down Sink Drains										
Check For Broken Furniture (Report/Schedule Maintenance)										
Light Bulbs Checked And None Functioning Bulbs Replaced										
Check Hardware, Door Stops And Lock Mechanisms										
Fire Exit Lights And Emergency Lights Checked & Functioning										
Test Carbon Monoxide Alarm And Replace Batteries If Required										
Test Smoke Detector Alarm And Replace Batteries If Required										
Paper Dispensers And Paper Towel Rolls Re-Stocked										
Soap Dispensers, Hand Sanitizers And Hand Gels Are Refilled										
Face Masks, Protective Gloves And Face Shields Re-Stocked										

CARE HOME COMMUNAL AREA CLEANING *Checklist*

Building	Location	Room Number	Area

Start Date & Time	Finnish Date & Time	Name	Signature

	Care Home Cleaning Tasks - Communal Area	M	T	W	T	F	S	S	Cleaned By	Checked By	Date/Ti
1	Clean And Sanitize All The Desks And Tables										
2	Clean And Sanitize All The Counter Tops And Surface Areas										
3	Wipe Down The Walls Wherever There Are Spills And Splashes										
4	Disinfect Touch Points, Light Switches And Other Switches										
5	Clean And Disinfect All Doors, Handles And Doorknobs										
6	Clean And Dust Door Frames, Remember To Dust The Tops										
7	Dust Light Fixtures & Shades With A Duster Or A Microfibre Cloth										
8	Clean And Wipe Mirrors Remove Fingerprints, Smears & Dirt										
9	Clean And Sanitize Over Chair Tables										
10	Clean And Polish Bookshelves, Remember To Dust The Top										
11	Remove, Wash And Clean Any Dirty Cups Or Glasses										
12	Remove, Wash And Clean Any Dirty Plates, Bowels Or Cutlery										
13	Clean And Sanitize Any Chairs, Seats And Benches										
14	Water Jugs (Washed Thoroughly Each Day & Re-Filled)										
15	Water Any Plants And Flowers										
16	Dust Plant Leafs (A Healthy Plant Needs To Be Clear Of Dust)										
17	Empty The Waste Baskets And Recycling Bins										
18	Clean And Disinfectant The Waste Bins And Recycling Bins										
19	Clean And Wipe Down Windowsills										
20	Spray Air Freshener This Keeps The Room Smelling Fresh										
21	Clean And Disinfect Cabinets And Units										
22	Clean And Sanitize Desk Accessories										
23	Replace Dirty Table Linen And Move To Laundry Room										
24	Polish Any Wooden Furniture And Hardwood Surfaces										
25	Clean Skirting Boards/Baseboards And Corners										
26	Clean And Polish Fireplace Mantelpiece And Surrounds										
27	Wipe Down Equipment & Sanitize Tea And Coffee Making Facilities										
28	Clean And Sanitize Telephones, Cords/Leads & All Touch Points										
29	Clean And Sanitize Walking Sticks And Any Other Walking Aids										

Care Home Cleaning Tasks - Communal Area	M	T	W	T	F	S	S	Cleaned By	Checked By	Date/Time
Dust Television, Top Sides And Back, TV Unit And TV Stand										
Clean TV Screen With Soft Damp Cloth (Use Water/Cleaner)										
Vacuum/Hoover Between Furniture And The Walls										
Clean And Sanitize All Wheelchairs										
Check For Broken Wheelchairs, Frames and Wheels										
Vacuum Under Furniture, Units, Tables And Cabinets										
Vacuum And Hoover The Carpets, Mats And Rugs										
Vacuum Furnishings, Cushions, Chairs, Sofas And Couches										
Steam Clean Carpets And Rugs										
Dust And Clean Any Picture Frames And Wall Art										
Clean & Check Contents Of Medicine Trolleys & Cupboards										
Clean & Vacuum The Desk Chair, Legs And Chair Wheels										
Wash And Clean Air Vents										
Dust Ceiling Fan Blades With Duster Or A Microfibre Cloth										
Wash And Clean Windows (Inside And Outside)										
Dust And Clean The Walls From Top To Bottom										
Clean Blinds (Dust The Blinds With A Damp Microfibre Cloth)										
Clean Curtains (Vacuum On A Low Setting Or Wash If Possible)										
Dust And Wash Radiator Covers										
Wash And Clean Ceiling Light Covers										
Clean & Vacuum Central Heating Units (Backs Of Radiators)										
Clean And Disinfect Any Handrails										
Clean And Sanitize Computer, Keyboard And Computer Mice										
Clean And Sanitize iPads, Tablets, Laptops & Mobile Phones										
Floors Mopped Clean With Cleaning Or Disinfecting Solution										
The Floors Are Swept And Free From Debris And Litter										
Clean Sliding Doors and Room Partitions										
Throw Away Outdated Newspapers, Magazines, Papers										
Check For Broken Furniture (Report/Schedule Maintenance)										
Light Bulbs Checked And None Functioning Bulbs Replaced										
Check Hardware, Door Stops And Lock Mechanisms										
Fire Exit Lights And Emergency Lights Checked & Functioning										
Test Carbon Monoxide Alarm And Replace Batteries If Required										
Test Smoke Detector Alarm And Replace Batteries If Required										
Paper Dispensers And Paper Towel Rolls Re-Stocked										
Soap Dispensers, Hand Sanitizers And Hand Gels Are Refilled										
Face Masks, Protective Gloves And Face Shields Re-Stocked										

CARE HOME TOILET & RESTROOM CLEANING *Checklis*

Building	Location	Room Number	Area

Start Date & Time	Finnish Date & Time	Name	Signature

	Care Home Cleaning Tasks - Toilet & Restroom	M	T	W	T	F	S	S	Cleaned By	Checked By	Date/Tin
1	Clean And Sanitize All The Counter Tops And Surface Areas										
2	Wipe Down The Walls Wherever There Are Spills And Splashes										
3	Disinfect Touch Points, Light Switches And Other Switches										
4	Clean And Disinfect All Doors, Handles And Doorknobs										
5	Clean And Dust Door Frames, Remember To Dust The Tops										
6	Dust Light Fixtures With A Duster Or A Microfibre Cloth										
7	Wall Mirrors Cleaned With Glass Cleaner										
8	Clean Any Bathroom Glasses And Cups										
9	Clean And Sanitize Any Chairs And Seats										
10	Empty The Waste Basket And Recycling Bin										
11	Clean And Disinfectant The Waste Bin And Recycling Bin										
12	Clean And Wipe Down Windowsills										
13	Spray Air Freshener This Keeps The Room Smelling Fresh										
14	Air/Odour Control Systems Are Filled And Operating Correctly										
15	Clean Skirting Boards/Baseboards And Corners										
16	Vacuum And Hoover Bath Mats, Shower Mats And Rugs										
17	Replace Bath Mats, Shower Mats And Rugs With Clean Ones										
18	Steam Clean Carpets And Rugs										
19	Hand Towels Replaced With Fresh Clean Ones										
20	Bath Towels Replaced With Fresh Clean Ones										
21	Face Towels Replaced With Fresh Clean Ones										
22	Electric Hand Dryers Cleaned, Disinfected & Operating Correctly										
23	Soap Dispensers, Sanitizers And Hand Gels Are Refilled										
24	Clean & Check Contents Of Medicine Trolleys & Cupboards										
25	Clean And Disinfect Any Handrails										
26	Sinks, Taps And Fixtures Cleaned And Disinfected										
27	Clean And Disinfect Cabinets And Units										
28	Feminine Hygiene Dispensers Re-Stocked										
29	Feminine Hygiene Bins/Containers Emptied And Cleared										

Care Home Cleaning Tasks - Toilet & Restroom	M	T	W	T	F	S	S	Cleaned By	Checked By	Date/Time
Clean & Vacuum Central Heating Units (Backs Of Radiators)										
Wash And Clean Ceiling Light Covers										
Toilet Roll Holders And Toilet Rolls Re-Stocked										
Toilet Roll Holders Cleaned And Disinfected										
Clean Inside The Toilets And Urinals With Disinfectant										
Toilet Seats Cleaned And Disinfected										
Clean Top Of Toilets Tanks, The Bases And Behind Toilets										
Urinal Handles Cleaned And Disinfected										
Urinal Screens Cleaned, Disinfected And Blocks Replaced										
Paper Dispensers And Paper Towel Rolls Re-Stocked										
Paper Dispensers And Paper Towel Roll Cleaned & Disinfected										
The Floors Are Swept And Free From Debris And Litter										
Floors Mopped Clean With Cleaning Or Disinfecting Solution										
Put Up Or Place Wet Floor Signs After Mopping Floors										
Showers And Shower Heads, Cleaned And Disinfected										
Soak Shower Heads										
Clean And Disinfect Glass Shower Doors/Outer Doors										
Clean Soap Scum From Shower Walls										
Clean Blinds (Dust The Blinds With A Damp Microfibre Cloth)										
Clean Curtains (Vacuum On A Low Setting Or Wash If Possible)										
Dust And Wash Radiator Covers										
Clean And Disinfect Commodes Between Each Use										
Clean And Disinfect Shower Chairs Between Each Use										
Bath Hoists Cleaned And Disinfected Between Each Use										
Scrub Tub/Bath, Polish Facets And Taps, Clean & Disinfected										
Toothbrush Holders And Soap Holders Cleaned										
Re-Place Shower Curtains With Clean Fresh Ones										
Wash And Clean Air Vents										
Thoroughly Clean Grout And Tiles										
Disinfect And Clean All The Walls From Top To Bottom										
Wash And Clean Windows (Inside And Outside)										
Unclog The Drains (Sink, Bath And Shower)										
Pour Drain Cleaner Down Sink, Shower & Bath Drains										
Floor Drains And Drain Covers Are Open And Free Of Debris										
Hair Dryers Cleaned And Disinfected And Operating Correctly										
Light Bulbs Checked And None Functioning Bulbs Replaced										
Check Hardware, Door Stops And Lock Mechanisms										

CARE HOME BEDROOM CLEANING *Checklist*

Building	Location	Room Number	Area

Start Date & Time	Finnish Date & Time	Name	Signature

	Care Home Cleaning Tasks - Bedrooms	M	T	W	T	F	S	S	Cleaned By	Checked By	Date/Ti
1	Clean And Sanitize All The Desks And Tables										
2	Clean And Sanitize All The Counter Tops And Surface Areas										
3	Wipe Down The Walls Wherever There Are Spills And Splashes										
4	Disinfect Touch Points, Light Switches And Other Switches										
5	Clean And Disinfect All Doors, Handles And Doorknobs										
6	Clean And Dust Door Frames, Remember To Dust The Tops										
7	Dust Light Fixtures With A Duster Or A Microfibre Cloth										
8	Clean & Wipe Mirrors Remove Fingerprints, Smears & Dirt										
9	Clean And Dust Bedside Cabinets										
10	Clean And Sanitize Over Chair Tables										
11	Clean And Sanitize Over Bed Tables										
12	Clean And Check Bed Frames										
13	Mattresses Hoovered And Cleaned With Disinfectant										
14	Clean And Polish Bookshelves, Remember To Dust The Top										
15	Remove, Wash And Clean Any Dirty Cups Or Glasses										
16	Remove, Wash And Clean Any Dirty Plates, Bowels Or Cutlery										
17	Clean And Sanitize Any Chairs And Seats										
18	Water Jug (Washed Thoroughly Each Day & Re-Filled)										
19	Water Any Plants And Flowers										
20	Dust Plant Leafs (A Healthy Plant Needs To Be Clear Of Dust)										
21	Empty The Waste Basket And Recycling Bin										
22	Clean And Disinfectant The Waste Bin And Recycling Bin										
23	Clean And Wipe Down Windowsills										
24	Spray Air Freshener This Keeps The Room Smelling Fresh										
25	Clean And Disinfect Cabinets And Units										
26	Clean And Sanitize Desk Accessories										
27	Replace Dirty Linen And Move To Laundry Room										
28	Polish Any Wooden Furniture And Hardwood Surfaces										
29	Clean Skirting Boards/Baseboards And Corners										

Care Home Cleaning Tasks - Bedrooms Continued	M	T	W	T	F	S	S	Cleaned By	Checked By	Date/Time
Dust Television, Top Sides And Back, TV Unit And TV Stand										
Clean TV Screen With Soft Damp Cloth (Use Water/Cleaner)										
Vacuum/Hoover Between Bedroom Furniture And The Walls										
Clean And Sanitize Resident's Personal Wheelchair										
Check For Broken Wheelchairs, Frames and Wheels										
Vacuum Under Furniture, Beds, Sofas and Dressers										
Vacuum And Hoover The Carpets, Mats And Rugs										
Vacuum Furnishings, Cushions, Chairs, Sofas And Couches										
Steam Clean Carpets And Rugs										
Dust And Clean Any Picture Frames And Photo Frames										
Ledges, Flat Surfaces And The Tops Of Wardrobes Dusted										
Clean & Check Contents Of Medicine Trolleys & Cupboards										
Clean And Sanitize Mobile Phone, Phone Case And Screen										
Clean & Vacuum The Desk Chair, Legs And Chair Wheels										
Wash And Clean Air Vents										
Dust Ceiling Fan Blades With Duster Or A Microfibre Cloth										
Wash And Clean Windows (Inside And Outside)										
Dust And Clean The Walls From Top To Bottom										
Clean Blinds (Dust The Blinds With A Damp Microfibre Cloth)										
Clean Curtains (Vacuum On A Low Setting Or Wash If Possible)										
Dust And Wash Radiator Covers										
Wash And Clean Ceiling Light Covers										
Clean & Vacuum Central Heating Units (Backs Of Radiators)										
Clean And Disinfect Any Handrails										
Hand Towels Replaced With Fresh Clean Ones										
Sink Wall Mirror Cleaned With Glass Cleaner										
Sinks, Taps And Fixtures Cleaned And Disinfected										
Pour Drain Cleaner Down Sink Drains										
Check For Broken Furniture (Report/Schedule Maintenance)										
Light Bulbs Checked And None Functioning Bulbs Replaced										
Check Hardware, Door Stops And Lock Mechanisms										
Fire Exit Lights And Emergency Lights Checked & Functioning										
Test Carbon Monoxide Alarm And Replace Batteries If Required										
Test Smoke Detector Alarm And Replace Batteries If Required										
Paper Dispensers And Paper Towel Rolls Re-Stocked										
Soap Dispensers, Hand Sanitizers And Hand Gels Are Refilled										
Face Masks, Protective Gloves And Face Shields Re-Stocked										

CARE HOME COMMUNAL AREA CLEANING *Checklist*

Building	Location	Room Number	Area

Start Date & Time	Finnish Date & Time	Name	Signature

	Care Home Cleaning Tasks - Communal Area	M	T	W	T	F	S	S	Cleaned By	Checked By	Date/Ti
1	Clean And Sanitize All The Desks And Tables										
2	Clean And Sanitize All The Counter Tops And Surface Areas										
3	Wipe Down The Walls Wherever There Are Spills And Splashes										
4	Disinfect Touch Points, Light Switches And Other Switches										
5	Clean And Disinfect All Doors, Handles And Doorknobs										
6	Clean And Dust Door Frames, Remember To Dust The Tops										
7	Dust Light Fixtures & Shades With A Duster Or A Microfibre Cloth										
8	Clean And Wipe Mirrors Remove Fingerprints, Smears & Dirt										
9	Clean And Sanitize Over Chair Tables										
10	Clean And Polish Bookshelves, Remember To Dust The Top										
11	Remove, Wash And Clean Any Dirty Cups Or Glasses										
12	Remove, Wash And Clean Any Dirty Plates, Bowels Or Cutlery										
13	Clean And Sanitize Any Chairs, Seats And Benches										
14	Water Jugs (Washed Thoroughly Each Day & Re-Filled)										
15	Water Any Plants And Flowers										
16	Dust Plant Leafs (A Healthy Plant Needs To Be Clear Of Dust)										
17	Empty The Waste Baskets And Recycling Bins										
18	Clean And Disinfectant The Waste Bins And Recycling Bins										
19	Clean And Wipe Down Windowsills										
20	Spray Air Freshener This Keeps The Room Smelling Fresh										
21	Clean And Disinfect Cabinets And Units										
22	Clean And Sanitize Desk Accessories										
23	Replace Dirty Table Linen And Move To Laundry Room										
24	Polish Any Wooden Furniture And Hardwood Surfaces										
25	Clean Skirting Boards/Baseboards And Corners										
26	Clean And Polish Fireplace Mantelpiece And Surrounds										
27	Wipe Down Equipment & Sanitize Tea And Coffee Making Facilities										
28	Clean And Sanitize Telephones, Cords/Leads & All Touch Points										
29	Clean And Sanitize Walking Sticks And Any Other Walking Aids										

Care Home Cleaning Tasks - Communal Area	M	T	W	T	F	S	S	Cleaned By	Checked By	Date/Time
Dust Television, Top Sides And Back, TV Unit And TV Stand										
Clean TV Screen With Soft Damp Cloth (Use Water/Cleaner)										
Vacuum/Hoover Between Furniture And The Walls										
Clean And Sanitize All Wheelchairs										
Check For Broken Wheelchairs, Frames and Wheels										
Vacuum Under Furniture, Units, Tables And Cabinets										
Vacuum And Hoover The Carpets, Mats And Rugs										
Vacuum Furnishings, Cushions, Chairs, Sofas And Couches										
Steam Clean Carpets And Rugs										
Dust And Clean Any Picture Frames And Wall Art										
Clean & Check Contents Of Medicine Trolleys & Cupboards										
Clean & Vacuum The Desk Chair, Legs And Chair Wheels										
Wash And Clean Air Vents										
Dust Ceiling Fan Blades With Duster Or A Microfibre Cloth										
Wash And Clean Windows (Inside And Outside)										
Dust And Clean The Walls From Top To Bottom										
Clean Blinds (Dust The Blinds With A Damp Microfibre Cloth)										
Clean Curtains (Vacuum On A Low Setting Or Wash If Possible)										
Dust And Wash Radiator Covers										
Wash And Clean Ceiling Light Covers										
Clean & Vacuum Central Heating Units (Backs Of Radiators)										
Clean And Disinfect Any Handrails										
Clean And Sanitize Computer, Keyboard And Computer Mice										
Clean And Sanitize iPads, Tablets, Laptops & Mobile Phones										
Floors Mopped Clean With Cleaning Or Disinfecting Solution										
The Floors Are Swept And Free From Debris And Litter										
Clean Sliding Doors and Room Partitions										
Throw Away Outdated Newspapers, Magazines, Papers										
Check For Broken Furniture (Report/Schedule Maintenance)										
Light Bulbs Checked And None Functioning Bulbs Replaced										
Check Hardware, Door Stops And Lock Mechanisms										
Fire Exit Lights And Emergency Lights Checked & Functioning										
Test Carbon Monoxide Alarm And Replace Batteries If Required										
Test Smoke Detector Alarm And Replace Batteries If Required										
Paper Dispensers And Paper Towel Rolls Re-Stocked										
Soap Dispensers, Hand Sanitizers And Hand Gels Are Refilled										
Face Masks, Protective Gloves And Face Shields Re-Stocked										

CARE HOME TOILET & RESTROOM CLEANING *Checklist*

Building	Location	Room Number	Area

Start Date & Time	Finnish Date & Time	Name	Signature

	Care Home Cleaning Tasks - Toilet & Restroom	M	T	W	T	F	S	S	Cleaned By	Checked By	Date/Ti
1	Clean And Sanitize All The Counter Tops And Surface Areas										
2	Wipe Down The Walls Wherever There Are Spills And Splashes										
3	Disinfect Touch Points, Light Switches And Other Switches										
4	Clean And Disinfect All Doors, Handles And Doorknobs										
5	Clean And Dust Door Frames, Remember To Dust The Tops										
6	Dust Light Fixtures With A Duster Or A Microfibre Cloth										
7	Wall Mirrors Cleaned With Glass Cleaner										
8	Clean Any Bathroom Glasses And Cups										
9	Clean And Sanitize Any Chairs And Seats										
10	Empty The Waste Basket And Recycling Bin										
11	Clean And Disinfectant The Waste Bin And Recycling Bin										
12	Clean And Wipe Down Windowsills										
13	Spray Air Freshener This Keeps The Room Smelling Fresh										
14	Air/Odour Control Systems Are Filled And Operating Correctly										
15	Clean Skirting Boards/Baseboards And Corners										
16	Vacuum And Hoover Bath Mats, Shower Mats And Rugs										
17	Replace Bath Mats, Shower Mats And Rugs With Clean Ones										
18	Steam Clean Carpets And Rugs										
19	Hand Towels Replaced With Fresh Clean Ones										
20	Bath Towels Replaced With Fresh Clean Ones										
21	Face Towels Replaced With Fresh Clean Ones										
22	Electric Hand Dryers Cleaned, Disinfected & Operating Correctly										
23	Soap Dispensers, Sanitizers And Hand Gels Are Refilled										
24	Clean & Check Contents Of Medicine Trolleys & Cupboards										
25	Clean And Disinfect Any Handrails										
26	Sinks, Taps And Fixtures Cleaned And Disinfected										
27	Clean And Disinfect Cabinets And Units										
28	Feminine Hygiene Dispensers Re-Stocked										
29	Feminine Hygiene Bins/Containers Emptied And Cleared										

Care Home Cleaning Tasks - Toilet & Restroom	M	T	W	T	F	S	S	Cleaned By	Checked By	Date/Time
Clean & Vacuum Central Heating Units (Backs Of Radiators)										
Wash And Clean Ceiling Light Covers										
Toilet Roll Holders And Toilet Rolls Re-Stocked										
Toilet Roll Holders Cleaned And Disinfected										
Clean Inside The Toilets And Urinals With Disinfectant										
Toilet Seats Cleaned And Disinfected										
Clean Top Of Toilets Tanks, The Bases And Behind Toilets										
Urinal Handles Cleaned And Disinfected										
Urinal Screens Cleaned, Disinfected And Blocks Replaced										
Paper Dispensers And Paper Towel Rolls Re-Stocked										
Paper Dispensers And Paper Towel Roll Cleaned & Disinfected										
The Floors Are Swept And Free From Debris And Litter										
Floors Mopped Clean With Cleaning Or Disinfecting Solution										
Put Up Or Place Wet Floor Signs After Mopping Floors										
Showers And Shower Heads, Cleaned And Disinfected										
Soak Shower Heads										
Clean And Disinfect Glass Shower Doors/Outer Doors										
Clean Soap Scum From Shower Walls										
Clean Blinds (Dust The Blinds With A Damp Microfibre Cloth)										
Clean Curtains (Vacuum On A Low Setting Or Wash If Possible)										
Dust And Wash Radiator Covers										
Clean And Disinfect Commodes Between Each Use										
Clean And Disinfect Shower Chairs Between Each Use										
Bath Hoists Cleaned And Disinfected Between Each Use										
Scrub Tub/Bath, Polish Facets And Taps, Clean & Disinfected										
Toothbrush Holders And Soap Holders Cleaned										
Re-Place Shower Curtains With Clean Fresh Ones										
Wash And Clean Air Vents										
Thoroughly Clean Grout And Tiles										
Disinfect And Clean All The Walls From Top To Bottom										
Wash And Clean Windows (Inside And Outside)										
Unclog The Drains (Sink, Bath And Shower)										
Pour Drain Cleaner Down Sink, Shower & Bath Drains										
Floor Drains And Drain Covers Are Open And Free Of Debris										
Hair Dryers Cleaned And Disinfected And Operating Correctly										
Light Bulbs Checked And None Functioning Bulbs Replaced										
Check Hardware, Door Stops And Lock Mechanisms										

IMPORTANT DATES AND EVENTS *Checklist*

Name: .... **Date:** ....

Event/Occasion: .... **Time:** ....

Location: .... **Phone:** ....

.... **Email:** ....

.... **Web:** ....

Name: .... **Date:** ....

Event/Occasion: .... **Time:** ....

Location: .... **Phone:** ....

.... **Email:** ....

.... **Web:** ....

Name: .... **Date:** ....

Event/Occasion: .... **Time:** ....

Location: .... **Phone:** ....

.... **Email:** ....

.... **Web:** ....

Name: .... **Date:** ....

Event/Occasion: .... **Time:** ....

Location: .... **Phone:** ....

.... **Email:** ....

.... **Web:** ....

Name: .... **Date:** ....

Event/Occasion: .... **Time:** ....

Location: .... **Phone:** ....

.... **Email:** ....

.... **Web:** ....

Name: .... **Date:** ....

Event/Occasion: .... **Time:** ....

Location: .... **Phone:** ....

.... **Email:** ....

.... **Web:** ....

IMPORTANT DATES AND EVENTS *Checklist*

ne:	....	**Date:**	....
t/Occasion:	....	**Time:**	....
ation:	....	**Phone:**	....
	....	**Email:**	....
	....	**Web:**	....

ne:	....	**Date:**	....
t/Occasion:	....	**Time:**	....
ation:	....	**Phone:**	....
	....	**Email:**	....
	....	**Web:**	....

ne:	....	**Date:**	....
t/Occasion:	....	**Time:**	....
ation:	....	**Phone:**	....
	....	**Email:**	....
	....	**Web:**	....

ne:	....	**Date:**	....
t/Occasion:	....	**Time:**	....
ation:	....	**Phone:**	....
	....	**Email:**	....
	....	**Web:**	....

ne:	....	**Date:**	....
t/Occasion:	....	**Time:**	....
ation:	....	**Phone:**	....
	....	**Email:**	....
	....	**Web:**	....

e:	....	**Date:**	....
t/Occasion:	....	**Time:**	....
ation:	....	**Phone:**	....
	....	**Email:**	....
	....	**Web:**	....

IMPORTANT DATES AND EVENTS *Checklist*

Name:

Event/Occasion:

Location:

Date:

Time:

Phone:

Email:

Web:

Name:

Event/Occasion:

Location:

Date:

Time:

Phone:

Email:

Web:

Name:

Event/Occasion:

Location:

Date:

Time:

Phone:

Email:

Web:

Name:

Event/Occasion:

Location:

Date:

Time:

Phone:

Email:

Web:

Name:

Event/Occasion:

Location:

Date:

Time:

Phone:

Email:

Web:

Name:

Event/Occasion:

Location:

Date:

Time:

Phone:

Email:

Web:

IMPORTANT DATES AND EVENTS *Checklist*

e:	Date:
t/Occasion:	Time:
tion:	Phone:
	Email:
	Web:

e:	Date:
t/Occasion:	Time:
tion:	Phone:
	Email:
	Web:

e:	Date:
t/Occasion:	Time:
tion:	Phone:
	Email:
	Web:

e:	Date:
t/Occasion:	Time:
tion:	Phone:
	Email:
	Web:

e:	Date:
t/Occasion:	Time:
tion:	Phone:
	Email:
	Web:

e:	Date:
t/Occasion:	Time:
tion:	Phone:
	Email:
	Web:

ESSENTIAL CARE HOME CONTACT *Details*

Name: ....

Company: ....

Address: ....

....

....

Phone: ....

Phone: ....

Email: ....

Email: ....

Web: ....

Name: ....

Company: ....

Address: ....

....

....

Phone: ....

Phone: ....

Email: ....

Email: ....

Web: ....

Name: ....

Company: ....

Address: ....

....

....

Phone: ....

Phone: ....

Email: ....

Email: ....

Web: ....

Name: ....

Company: ....

Address: ....

....

....

Phone: ....

Phone: ....

Email: ....

Email: ....

Web: ....

Name: ....

Company: ....

Address: ....

....

....

Phone: ....

Phone: ....

Email: ....

Email: ....

Web: ....

Name: ....

Company: ....

Address: ....

....

Phone: ....

Phone: ....

Email: ....

Email: ....

Web: ....

ESSENTIAL CARE HOME CONTACT *Details*

e: _____
pany: _____
ess: _____
_____
_____

Phone: _____
Phone: _____
Email: _____
Email: _____
Web: _____

---

e: _____
pany: _____
ess: _____
_____
_____

Phone: _____
Phone: _____
Email: _____
Email: _____
Web: _____

---

e: _____
pany: _____
ess: _____
_____
_____

Phone: _____
Phone: _____
Email: _____
Email: _____
Web: _____

---

e: _____
pany: _____
ess: _____
_____
_____

Phone: _____
Phone: _____
Email: _____
Email: _____
Web: _____

---

e: _____
pany: _____
ess: _____
_____
_____

Phone: _____
Phone: _____
Email: _____
Email: _____
Web: _____

---

e: _____
pany: _____
ess: _____
_____

Phone: _____
Phone: _____
Email: _____
Email: _____
Web: _____

CARE HOME TO DO TASKS *Checklist*

Name:........................... **Location:**................... **Date:**.............. **Week No:**............

HIGH PRIORITY - To Do List... ☆☑ ☆☑ ☆☑	DATE	DO
1.	....	◯
2.	....	◯
3.	....	◯
4.	....	◯
5.	....	◯
6.	....	◯
7.	....	◯
8.	....	◯
9.	....	◯
10.	....	◯

MEDIUM PRIORITY - To Do List... ☆☑ ☆☑	DATE	DO
1.	....	◯
2.	....	◯
3.	....	◯
4.	....	◯
5.	....	◯
6.	....	◯
7.	....	◯
8.	....	◯
9.	....	◯
10.	....	◯

LOW PRIORITY - To Do List... ☆☑	DATE	DO
1.	....	◯
2.	....	◯
3.	....	◯
4.	....	◯
5.	....	◯
6.	....	◯
7.	....	◯
8.	....	◯
9.	....	◯
10.	....	◯

CARE HOME TO DO TASKS *Checklist*

Name:............................ Location:.................................... Date:.................... Week No:....................

HIGH PRIORITY - To Do List... ⭐⭐⭐	DATE	DONE
		◯
		◯
		◯
		◯
		◯
		◯
		◯
		◯
		◯
		◯

MEDIUM PRIORITY - To Do List... ⭐⭐	DATE	DONE
		◯
		◯
		◯
		◯
		◯
		◯
		◯
		◯
		◯
		◯
		◯

LOW PRIORITY - To Do List... ⭐	DATE	DONE
		◯
		◯
		◯
		◯
		◯
		◯
		◯
		◯
		◯
		◯

CARE HOME TO DO TASKS *Checklist*

Name: .... **Location:** .... **Date:** .... **Week No:** ....

HIGH PRIORITY - To Do List... ⭐⭐⭐	DATE	DC

1. ....
2. ....
3. ....
4. ....
5. ....
6. ....
7. ....
8. ....
9. ....
10. ....

MEDIUM PRIORITY - To Do List... ⭐⭐	DATE	DC

1. ....
2. ....
3. ....
4. ....
5. ....
6. ....
7. ....
8. ....
9. ....
10. ....

LOW PRIORITY - To Do List... ⭐	DATE	DC

1. ....
2. ....
3. ....
4. ....
5. ....
6. ....
7. ....
8. ....
9. ....
10. ....

CARE HOME TO DO TASKS *Checklist*

e:............................ **Location:**............................ **Date:**............................ **Week No:**............................

HIGH PRIORITY - To Do List... ☆ ☆ ☆	DATE	DONE
		◯
		◯
		◯
		◯
		◯
		◯
		◯
		◯
		◯
		◯

MEDIUM PRIORITY - To Do List... ☆ ☆	DATE	DONE
		◯
		◯
		◯
		◯
		◯
		◯
		◯
		◯
		◯
		◯

LOW PRIORITY - To Do List... ☆	DATE	DONE
		◯
		◯
		◯
		◯
		◯
		◯
		◯
		◯
		◯
		◯

ESSENTIAL CLEANING INVENTORY *Checklist*

Date	Establishment/Location	Counted By

SKU/Product No	Product/Description	Quantity	Price	Reorder Da

ESSENTIAL CLEANING INVENTORY *Checklist*

Date	Establishment/Location	Counted By

SKU/Product No	Product/Description	Quantity	Price	Reorder Date

ESSENTIAL CLEANING INVENTORY *Checklist*

Date	Establishment/Location	Counted By

SKU/Product No	Product/Description	Quantity	Price	Reorder Da

ESSENTIAL CLEANING INVENTORY *Checklist*

Date	Establishment/Location	Counted By

SKU/Product No	Product/Description	Quantity	Price	Reorder Date

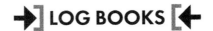 **LOG BOOKS**

"Thank you for being an exceptional customer."

We hope that your book exceeded your expectations?

Creating notebooks is what we do!

We **GO<AllOUT** when it comes to designing books.

If you have any ideas for notebooks, log books, planners, journals diaries, work or composition books, we would love to hear from you.

And maybe we can make those ideas come to life!

Additional pages?
New features or sections creating?
Other book sizes?
Any covers or page design ideas?
Any industries or sectors you require notebooks for?

Please email any book suggestions to:

sales@**ALLOUT**GROUP.co.uk

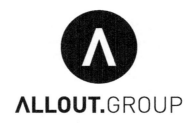

ALLOUT.GROUP

www.**ALLOUT**GROUP.co.uk

Printed in Great Britain
by Amazon

48990863R00112